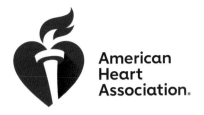

American Heart Association.

Basic Life Support

INSTRUCTOR MANUAL

© 2020 American Heart Association
ISBN 978-1-61669-769-3
Printed in the United States of America

First American Heart Association Printing October 2020
10 9 8 7 6 5 4 3 2 1

Acknowledgments

The American Heart Association thanks the following people for their contributions to the development of this manual: Jose G. Cabañas, MD, MPH; Jeanette Previdi, MPH, RN; Matthew Douma, RN; Bryan Fischberg, NRP; Sonni Logan, MSN, RN, CEN, CVN, CPEN; Mary Elizabeth Mancini, RN, PhD, NE-BC; Randy Wax, MD, MEd; Sharon T. Wilson, PhD, RN, FCN; Brenda D. Schoolfield; and the AHA BLS Project Team.

 To find out about any updates or corrections to this text, visit **www.heart.org/courseupdates**.

Contents

Contents

BLS Instructor Resources

These resources are available on the AHA Instructor Network at **www.ahainstructornetwork.org**.

Precourse Materials

Equipment List

Sample Precourse Letter to Students (Classroom Course)

Sample Precourse Letter to Students (HeartCode BLS)

Sample BLS Course Agenda With Optional Lessons

Sample BLS Renewal Course Agenda Without Optional Lessons

Sample HeartCode BLS Agenda With Optional Lessons

Sample HeartCode BLS Agenda Without Optional Lessons

Course Materials

Adult CPR and AED Skills Testing Checklist

Adult CPR and AED Skills Testing Critical Skills Descriptors

Infant CPR Skills Testing Checklist

Infant CPR Skills Testing Critical Skills Descriptors

Team Dynamics Diagram

Summary of High-Quality CPR Components for BLS Providers

BLS Lesson Plans

BLS Renewal Lesson Plans

HeartCode BLS Lesson Plans

Part 1

General Concepts

About This Instructor Manual

We have reorganized our instructor manuals to provide an introductory section that discusses the science and educational principles of resuscitation training as well as the basic logistics for conducting any American Heart Association (AHA) course. For new instructors, Part 1 provides essential and practical tools to help launch them as AHA Instructors. For more seasoned instructors, Part 1 offers insights into the science and educational principles that go into the design of all AHA courses. Although some of this information applies mostly to the AHA advanced resuscitation courses, Basic Life Support (BLS) Instructors may find it useful. The remaining Parts of this instructor manual cover course-specific information.

Critical Role of the Instructor

The ultimate goal of AHA courses is to improve outcomes for people with cardiovascular disease, especially those who need cardiopulmonary resuscitation (CPR) or emergency cardiovascular care (ECC). AHA Instructors have a unique opportunity to impact the survival of real people by helping to enhance student skills through learning and practice. Instructors should use the educational design of ECC courses to simulate events that are as close to real emergencies as possible. In this way, AHA courses can prepare students to function optimally for their next emergency.

As an AHA Instructor, your role is to help your students by

Demonstrating effective case management consistent with the current AHA Guidelines for CPR and ECC

- Modeling high-quality principles of care
- Facilitating discussions with a focus on desired outcome
- Listening to students' responses and providing feedback to ensure that they understand the learning concepts
- Observing students' actions and coaching them as necessary
- Providing positive or corrective feedback
- Managing discussions and simulations to optimize classroom time and maximize learning
- Leading, modeling, and promoting prebriefing sessions before each simulation and structured debriefing sessions after each simulation

Some AHA Instructors will also teach blended-learning courses. These courses combine eLearning, in which a student completes part of the course online, with a hands-on instructor-led session. You'll learn more about blended-learning courses later in this manual.

Instructor Needs and Resources

Science Update Information

Science and education updates occur periodically. The AHA provides the following resources so that you can access these updates as they are released:

- The AHA Instructor Network, which includes the *ECC Beat*; for instructions on how to access, visit **www.ahainstructornetwork.org**
- The AHA website (**cpr.heart.org**)

For full details of all changes that were made to the resuscitation guidelines, the AHA strongly recommends that each instructor access the guidelines, available at **eccguidelines.heart.org**.

Instructor Network

The AHA provides the Instructor Network as a resource to instructors. Here, instructors can access up-to-date resources and reference information about the AHA ECC programs and science.

AHA Instructor Registration

www.ahainstructornetwork.org

All AHA Instructors are required to register with the AHA to be aligned with a Training Center. For instructions on how to register, visit **www.ahainstructornetwork.org**. Alignment must be approved by that Training Center before access to content is available. Acceptance of the user agreement is required during registration.

Once registered and approved, you will receive an instructor identification number. This number will be placed on your instructor card and is the same for all disciplines. This number stays the same if you change Training Centers. It is used on all course completions cards for classes that you teach.

The AHA reserves the right to delete or deny alignments on the Instructor Network.

Course Planning and Support Materials

Before teaching a classroom course or hands-on session, please take the time to read and review in detail the instructor manual and lesson plans, provider manual and any additional student resources, and videos. Your preparation is key to a successful and rewarding teaching experience.

As you view the videos and the lesson plans (Parts 5 and 6), note how the course is organized and the expectations for you and the students. Make notes on your lesson plans as needed.

This important preparation will enable you to teach the course more effectively and anticipate what you will need to do as the course unfolds. This is especially true for those parts of the course that require you to organize the students for practice or testing, present the video to give information, facilitate discussions, distribute equipment, conduct debriefings, and give exams or hands-on tests.

Notice of Courses

 For US-based instructors aligned with the AHA Instructor Network, the AHA offers the My Courses tool, where instructors can enter and maintain the classes they offer to the general public. These are displayed to customers searching for scheduled classes on the AHA's CPR and First Aid website, **cpr.heart.org**. Before entering classes, check with your Training Center to determine what policies that center may have about instructors entering their classes. As an instructor, you can still add your classes for display through My Courses even if your Training Center is not participating in listing through My Courses.

For instructors based outside the United States, inform your International Training Center of courses open to the public so that they can send inquiries for classes to you.

Ordering Materials

 As an instructor, you can order books and other support materials through your Training Center or directly from the AHA at **ShopCPR.Heart.org**. There are also distributors available for AHA Instructors outside the United States (**https://international.heart.org/en/how-to-buy**). However, only a Training Center Coordinator can order course completion cards. Work with your Training Center Coordinator to ensure that your students receive their cards.

Copyright of AHA Materials

The AHA owns the copyright to AHA books and other training materials. These materials may not be copied, in whole or in part, without the prior written consent of the AHA.

 For more information and to request permission to reprint, copy, or use portions of ECC textbooks or other materials, go to **copyright.heart.org**.

Smoking Policy

The Training Center must prohibit smoking in classrooms and training facilities during all AHA ECC training programs.

Course Completion Cards

Only a Training Center Coordinator, or another authorized Training Center representative designated by the Training Center Coordinator, can use the confidential security code to order course completion cards (eCard or printed) for approved disciplines. The Training Center Coordinator should keep this code confidential. Training Center Coordinators cannot order course completion cards without this code.

The Training Center Coordinator has final responsibility to the AHA for the security code. The Training Center Coordinator must notify ECC Customer Support immediately if the security code is suspected as lost, stolen, disclosed, or used without authorization.

The AHA may change the code if deemed necessary to maintain the confidentiality of the code.

Misuse of the confidential security code could result in termination of the Training Center Agreement.

 For more information on course completion cards, refer to the ECC Course Card Reference Guide on the Instructor Network and at **cpr.heart.org**.

Course Equipment

All AHA ECC courses require that manikins and equipment allow demonstration of the core skills (eg, airway management, correct hand placement, compression depth, chest recoil). The AHA requires the use of an instrumented directive feedback device or manikin in all AHA courses that teach the skills of adult CPR.

The AHA neither endorses nor recommends a particular brand of manikin or other equipment. The decision on which brand or model of equipment to use is the responsibility of the Training Center.

You can find a detailed equipment list for your course or hands-on session in Part 2 of this instructor manual.

High-Fidelity vs Low-Fidelity Simulation

Simulators have been used to teach BLS for decades. They give students the opportunity to practice and improve the clinical skills needed for resuscitating real patients.

Because of improvements in technology, healthcare professionals can more easily observe pathophysiologic signs. The variety of simulators has expanded considerably. Some are as simple and old-fashioned as using an orange to practice intramuscular injections. Others are more sophisticated, such as computer-guided mechanical devices that make practicing specific procedures look and feel more real. Improved plastics have made task trainers (eg, airway practice models) more versatile and realistic, and many manikins have lifelike features and enhancements.

While the term *high fidelity* has been used as a synonym for high technology, fidelity actually refers to the level of realism as this relates to specific learning objectives. Thus, high fidelity implies a very realistic simulation, while low fidelity implies that the student must use his or her imagination to fill in the gaps. These definitions are based on the experience of the student rather than on the device itself.

While advanced technology and high-fidelity simulation are appealing and may result in higher student satisfaction, they increase costs substantially without necessarily enhancing learning compared with more basic simulators. In fact, none of the available products are truly realistic compared with real human beings.

You may find high-fidelity manikins useful for teamwork and skills integration, but it is not certain which specific aspects of the scenario are improved by a higher degree of realism. Having a relevant case and setting for students—or matching the equipment to what the students use in their practices—may be more important than a high-fidelity manikin for translating the learning process to clinical practice. As an instructor, you can tailor your approach by using the resources available to create a high-fidelity environment that both satisfies students and achieves the desired learning objectives.

Feedback devices can accurately measure rate, depth, and recoil of compressions and rate and volume of ventilation. This feedback should be used throughout the course and for testing so that students are able to practice until they can do it without having to think about it (ie, automatically). Because you are trying to build automaticity, it is important for students to perform these skills correctly and consistently and for Team Leaders and team members to recognize correct performance by others.

Infection Control

It is your responsibility as an instructor to ensure that a safe, clean environment is maintained in your class. Inform your students in advance that training sessions involve close physical contact with manikins and that they will be close to other students.

In your welcome letter that is sent with course materials, tell students not to attend class if they know they have an infectious disease, feel sick, or have open sores or cuts on their hands, mouth, or areas around their mouth. Participants and instructors should postpone CPR training if they are in the active stages of an infectious disease or have reason to believe they have been exposed to an infectious disease.

Equipment and Manikin Cleaning

To reduce the risk of potential disease transmission, all manikins and training equipment need to be thoroughly cleaned after each class. Manikins used for CPR practice and testing require special actions to be taken between each student. The AHA strongly recommends that you follow manufacturers' recommendations for manikin use and maintenance. In the absence of manufacturers' recommendations, the following guidelines may be used during and after class:

During Class
- Students and instructors should practice good hygiene with proper handwashing techniques.
- When individual protective face shields are used, continue to follow all decontamination recommendations listed for cleaning manikins during and after a course. In addition, to reduce the risks to each user for exposure to contaminants, ensure that all students consistently place the same side of the face shield on the manikin during use.
- If you are not using face shields during the course, clean the manikins after use by each student with a manikin wipe that has an antiseptic with 70% ethyl alcohol.
    - Open the packet, and take out and unfold the manikin wipe.
    - Rub the manikin's mouth and nose vigorously with the wipe.
    - Wrap the wipe snugly over the mouth and nose.
    - Keep the wipe in place for 30 seconds.
    - Dry the manikin's face with a clean paper towel or something similar.
    - Continue with the ventilation practice.

After Class
- Take apart the manikins as directed by the manufacturer. Anyone taking apart and decontaminating manikins should wear protective gloves and wash their hands when finished.
- As soon as possible after each class, clean any part of the manikin that comes into contact with potentially infectious body fluids during training to prevent contaminants from drying on manikin surfaces.
- If manikins are stored for more than 24 hours before cleaning, follow these steps:
    - Wash all surfaces, reusable protective face shields, and pocket masks thoroughly with warm, soapy water and brushes.
    - Moisten all surfaces with a sodium hypochlorite solution having at least 500 ppm free available chlorine (one quarter cup of liquid household bleach per gallon of tap water) for 10 minutes. Make this solution fresh for each class and discard after each use. Using a concentration higher than one quarter cup has not been proven to be more effective and may discolor the manikins.
    - Rinse all surfaces with fresh water and air dry before storing.

- Because some manufacturers have recommendations for cleaning manikin parts in a dishwasher, check with the manufacturer of the manikins being used to determine if this is an acceptable method. Some manikin materials could be damaged in a dishwasher.
- Replace disposable airway equipment at the end of each class.
- Clean manikin clothing and the manikin carrying case periodically or when soiled.
- Maintain other equipment used in class according to hospital policy. Wipe surfaces touched by students with antiseptic solution.

Course Materials

Templates

As a registered instructor, you can log in to your account to find templates for letters, forms, and other materials to help you prepare to teach the course. You will need to customize some of these materials, including the precourse letter, which tells students what they need to do to prepare for the course or hands-on session.

Lesson Plans

All AHA ECC instructor manuals include lesson plans that are intended to

- Help you as an instructor to facilitate your courses
- Ensure consistency from course to course
- Help you focus on the main objectives for each lesson
- Explain your responsibilities during the course

Your lesson plans were created to be used before and during courses and during skills practice and testing sessions, as noted in Table 1.

Table 1. How to Use Lesson Plans

When	How to use
Before the course	Review your lesson plans, making notes of anything you want to emphasize on the basis of your students' roles and environment. • Identify objectives for each lesson. • Define your role for each lesson plan. • Gather the resources needed for each lesson.
During the course	• Follow each lesson plan as you conduct the course. • Remind students what each video segment covers. • Make sure you have all the resources, equipment, and supplies ready for each lesson. • Help all students achieve the objectives identified for each lesson. • Encourage students to work in teams and to help each other. • Create an atmosphere that encourages peak performance and improvement that will carry over into clinical practice.
During practice before a skills test	A student may have a question about a certain part of skills they will be tested on. The lesson plans serve as a resource for you when answering those questions.

Using the Provider Manual

Students must have their own copy of the current provider manual to read before and to use as a resource during and after the course. The lesson plans tell you when to refer students to specific sections of the provider manual during the course.

The provider manual is designed for individual use and is an integral part of the student's education. Students may reuse their manuals during renewals or updates until new science guidelines are published.

Students taking a blended-learning course have access to the provider manual and other reference materials within the online portion. They may access the reference materials for up to 2 years from the date they activate their online portion. Students should be allowed to bring electronic devices into the classroom to access these electronic materials.

Tailoring to the Audience

Determining Course Specifics

Before you teach a course, determine the course specifics:

- Student audience
- Number of students
- Special needs or local protocols
- Room requirements
- Course equipment

Details specific for the type of course or hands-on session that you will be conducting are located in Part 3.

Course Flexibility

The AHA allows instructors to tailor their courses to meet audience-specific needs. One example of this course flexibility is local protocol discussions built into some of the lessons. For specific examples, refer to Part 2.

Any changes to the course are in addition to the basic course contents as outlined in this manual and will add to the length of the course. Instructors may not delete course lessons or course components. Any additions or alterations to the course must be specifically identified as non-AHA material (refer to the Non-AHA Content section). Some evidence suggests that adding content to the course may actually decrease learning and retention. Although it is not considered a best practice to insert additional material into this course, instructors may add related topics, as long as none of the required lessons or course content is eliminated or shortened.

Non-AHA Content

As an instructor, you can best serve your students when you can adapt to meet the needs of a specific audience. If you find that your students will be better served by adding location-specific information, equipment, or specialty-specific content and you plan to discuss that non-AHA content in class or distribute handouts, follow these rules:

- None of the required AHA lessons or course content can be eliminated or shortened.
- Any changes to the course are in addition to the basic content as outlined in your instructor manual.
- Adding additional content will add time to the course.
- Additional topics or information should be covered at the *beginning or end* of the course to avoid disrupting the flow of the required lessons.
- Any location-specific protocols or procedures that do not comply with AHA processes (eg, substituting new medications, specialized techniques) should be identified to the audience as *location-specific*.
- Any non-AHA content must be identified as *not approved or reviewed by the AHA*, and the source of the information must be provided to the students.
- Supplementary materials that you use need to be approved by the Lead Instructor or the Course Director for advanced courses, as well as by your Training Center Coordinator.
- A copy of a revised agenda and any print material shared in class must be part of the permanent course file.
- Your students cannot be tested on non-AHA content. If they complete the AHA-defined course completion requirements, they must be issued an AHA course completion card.

Students With Special Needs

- The AHA does not provide advice to Training Centers on Americans With Disabilities Act requirements or any other laws, rules, or regulations. Training Centers must determine accommodations necessary to comply with applicable laws. The AHA recommends consultation with legal counsel.

- A student must be able to successfully complete all course completion requirements to receive a course completion card. Reasonable accommodations may be made, such as manikin positioning, use of a text reader, or reading the exam to the student.

- If a student is unable to successfully complete skills testing because of a disability, he or she should be given written documentation of class attendance, with a listing of what testing was not successfully completed.

- Advisor: BLS course completion cards accommodate students who pass the cognitive portion of the HeartCode® BLS Course but cannot perform the physical skills of CPR. By successfully advising others how to perform CPR and use an automated external defibrillator (AED), HeartCode BLS students with disabilities can receive an Advisor: BLS card. Students should check to make sure that their workplaces will accept these cards. Advisor: BLS cards are available exclusively to authorized Training Centers for issuance in accordance with AHA policy.

Implementing Resuscitation Education Science in Training

According to research reviewed in the 2018 AHA Scientific Statement "Resuscitation Education Science: Educational Strategies to Improve Outcomes From Cardiac Arrest," providers' skills can begin to decay only weeks after taking standardized resuscitation courses, which can lead to poor clinical care and survival outcomes for cardiac arrest patients. The Resuscitation Education Statement presented evidence supporting the following strategies to improve how well providers learn and retain these critical skills.

- Mastery learning: To increase the likelihood that a student will truly learn key resuscitation skills, have students practice until they demonstrate mastery. AHA courses are designed to give students time to practice with video demonstration, scenarios, and group activities. As an AHA Instructor, your role is to provide the feedback and coaching to make students' practice time meaningful and effective.

- Perfect practice makes perfect: Use a mastery learning model that requires students to demonstrate key skills, and set a minimum passing standard for mastery. Video demonstrations in AHA courses allow students to observe accurate and consistent resuscitation skills and to practice with the video and in group scenarios. Give students time to practice until they are comfortable with the skills and feel ready to take the skills test.

- Measuring performance to motivate students: Set performance standards on the basis of observable behaviors. Determine the most important measures for patient outcomes and process standards such as time, accuracy, and best practices. The skills testing checklists in all AHA courses define the passing standard for critical skills and allow instructors to measure and document student performance.

- Deliberate practice: Use skill repetition paired with feedback and exercises, known as *deliberate practice*, to teach behaviors that are difficult to master or should be performed automatically.

- Use of overlearning to improve retention: Train students beyond the minimum standard, known as *overlearning*, for behaviors that are likely to decay and would require effort to retrain someone to a level of mastery.

- Spaced learning: Students who participate in more frequent, shorter learning sessions have a better chance of retaining new knowledge and procedures. Strategies like eLearning, rolling refresher events, and other ways to increase learning outside of scheduled training can reinforce training after the class. Resuscitation Quality Improvement® is an example of low-dose, high-frequency training that providers can use to regularly practice skills and reinforce learning at their workplace. Instructors may offer periodic skills refreshers between course events.

- Contextual learning: Training that applies directly to students' scope of practice can engage students and make them eager to expand their expertise. Ensure that team composition, roles, and contexts are right for each group activity, and consider implementing appropriate levels of stress and cognitive load.

- Prebriefing, feedback, and debriefing:
  - Prebriefing: Briefing before a learning event creates a safe environment for students by setting their expectations. Prebriefing builds rapport between instructor and student, which can make students more receptive to feedback after the event.
  - Using data in feedback and debriefing: Students need performance data to improve. This includes data from instructors, other students, and devices.
  - Debriefing tools: Debriefing tools or scripts improve instructors' debriefing effectiveness by providing direction and content that is focused on improving learning outcomes.

- Assessment: Assessment of student competence is a critical part of developing efficient resuscitation teams. Plan for various, high-quality assessments throughout each course to get a broader picture of each student's knowledge and skills.

- Innovative educational strategies: New methods of accessing up-to-date information can improve laypeople's willingness to act, provider performance, and survival rates. For example, gamified learning can improve engagement, and social media delivers information quickly to large audiences.
- Faculty development: Initial instructor training is crucial, but empowering instructors to commit to lifelong learning creates a culture of training excellence, inspires students, and enhances the classroom experience.
- Knowledge translation and implementation strategies: The best evidence evaluation won't improve patient survival if providers aren't able to apply the knowledge gained to clinical practice. According to the Resuscitation Education Statement, improving methods for translating scientific knowledge into clinical practice is an ongoing field of study that could save more lives than a new breakthrough in managing cardiac arrest. AHA courses teach resuscitation skills as well as team skills and use tools like debriefing so that students learn not only how to perform the critical skills but how to assess and analyze behaviors in real resuscitation events to help their teams improve performance.

Importance of High-Quality CPR

High-quality CPR, comprising manual chest compressions and ventilation, is the foundation of lifesaving resuscitation for cardiac arrest victims. Maintaining blood flow to the heart and brain is the first priority, ahead of other interventions, such as administering medications. Individuals and teams should focus on maintaining cardiac output at all times during an attempted resuscitation for cardiac arrest.

Too often, CPR either is not performed or is performed with too many interruptions during both out-of-hospital and in-hospital arrests. Studies of CPR skills retention have shown patterns of significant erosion of CPR skills in the days, weeks, and months after CPR training. CPR should be performed in real time with an audiovisual feedback device guiding each student's performance in all learning stations where CPR is required. This is critical for a high-performance team. In addition, chest compression fraction (CCF), the proportion of time that chest compressions are performed during a cardiac arrest, should drive increased performance in learning stations and cannot be measured unless compressions are conducted in real time. Ventilation should also be timed or have real-time audiovisual feedback to help ensure optimal performance. This is true in practice, in testing, and in real-life emergencies.

All students will have the opportunity to practice high-quality CPR and then to demonstrate these lifesaving skills during the course assessment.

Components of high-quality CPR for adult cardiac arrest victims include the following:

- Push hard (at least 2 inches [5 cm]), using an automated feedback device to assist with performance improvement.
- Push fast, compressing at a rate of 100 to 120 per minute.
- Minimize interruptions in compressions to less than 10 seconds.
- Achieve a CCF that is ideally greater than 80%.
- Allow for complete chest recoil between compressions (ie, do not lean on the chest between compressions).
- Avoid excessive ventilation, delivering breaths over 1 second that produce visible chest rise.
- Switch compressors about every 2 minutes or earlier if fatigued.

High-Performance Teamwork

With resuscitation teams, high-performance teamwork is a critical element of providing high-quality CPR and increasing survival rates. Resuscitation skills competency is most often verified on an individual basis despite the fact that successful patient outcome from cardiac arrest depends on a team. Students will learn about high-performance teamwork and will practice it in the classroom.

High-performance teams effectively incorporate timing, quality, coordination, and administration of the appropriate procedures during a cardiac arrest (Figure 1). These 4 key areas of focus include the following specifics:

- **Timing:** time to first compression, time to first shock, CCF ideally greater than 80%, minimizing preshock pause, and early emergency medical services (EMS) response time
- **Quality:** rate, depth, complete recoil; minimizing interruptions; switching compressors every 2 minutes or sooner if fatigued; avoiding excessive ventilation; and always using a feedback device
- **Coordination:** team dynamics; team members working together, proficient in their roles
- **Administration:** leadership, measurement, CQI, number of participating code team members

Teams function differently in different facilities and in all out-of-hospital settings. Knowing the policies and procedures and the local protocols of your classroom audience is essential to instructor preparation.

Figure 1. Key areas of focus for high-performance teams to increase survival rates.

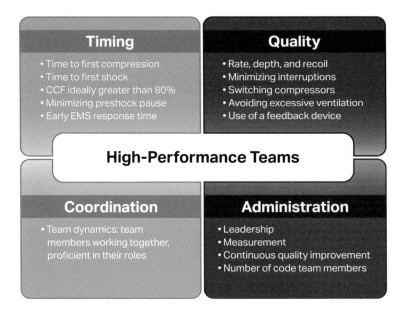

The Role of a CPR Coach in a Resuscitation Team

When caring for a cardiac arrest victim, the resuscitation team must perform many important tasks. Efficiently coordinating these tasks is critical to improving patient outcome. The Team Leader is typically responsible for monitoring the performance of BLS skills in addition to overseeing many other critical tasks. Coordinating so much at once is difficult and can lead to delays and errors in treatment.

For these reasons, many resuscitation teams now include the role of CPR Coach. The CPR Coach supports performance of high-quality BLS skills, allowing the Team Leader to focus on other aspects of clinical care. Studies have shown that resuscitation teams with a CPR Coach perform higher-quality CPR with higher CCF and shorter pause durations compared with teams that don't use a CPR Coach.

The CPR Coach does not need to be a separate role; they can be blended into the current responsibilities of the Monitor/Defibrillator. The CPR Coach's responsibilities begin with the start of CPR. A primary focus is to coach team members in performing high-quality BLS skills and help them minimize pauses in chest compressions. Here is a brief summary of specific responsibilities:

Coordinate the start of CPR: As soon as the patient is identified as pulseless, the CPR Coach prompts action by saying, "I am the CPR Coach. There is no pulse, so let's start compressions." The CPR Coach then prepares the environment to optimize compressions. This may include lowering the bed and bed rails, getting a step stool, or rolling the victim to place the backboard and defibrillator pads. These actions help prevent Compressor fatigue and ensure high-quality compressions.

Coach to improve the quality of chest compressions and ventilation: The CPR Coach does the following to help improve the quality of chest compressions and ventilation:

- Convey objective data from a CPR feedback device to help the Compressor improve performance. Team members' visual assessment of CPR quality is commonly inaccurate.
- Coach performance of compressions (ie, depth, rate, and chest recoil) and ventilation (ie, ventilation rate, volume and if needed, compression-to-ventilation ratio).
- State the specific midrange targets to help team members perform compressions and ventilation within the recommended range (eg, tell them to compress at a rate of 110/min instead of a rate between 100 and 120/min).
- Give corrective feedback and reinforce positive performance of CPR skills with specific acknowledgment (eg, good job with compression depth).

Coordinate provider switches and defibrillation: The CPR Coach helps minimize the length of pauses during provider switches and defibrillation. The goal is to pause for less than 5 seconds.

Here is an example of a CPR Coach's dialogue: "Team Leader, we have 30 seconds until the next pulse check. Next Compressor, please come stand by the current Compressor. I'll precharge the defibrillator, and then I'll give a 5 second countdown. The Compressor will stop compressions at 1 second. Then, the Compressors will switch and hover over the chest. We'll check a pulse, and the Team Leader will assess the rhythm. If it's a shockable rhythm, we'll shock immediately and then resume compressions."

Coordinate the placement of an advanced airway: The CPR Coach coordinates the placement of an advanced airway to minimize interruptions in compressions. First, the CPR Coach ensures that the Team Leader and Airway provider have a shared understanding: "My understanding is that we'll attempt intubation without stopping compressions. If that doesn't work, we can pause for up to 10 seconds for the intubation attempt. Is that correct?" Then, the CPR Coach announces the start of the intubation attempt and coordinates a pause if needed. Once the pause duration reaches 10 seconds, the CPR Coach directs the Compressor to start compressions again.

Instructor Tips

- Any healthcare professional can be a CPR Coach. This person must have a current BLS Provider card, understand the responsibilities of a CPR Coach, and demonstrate the ability to coach Compressors and Airway providers effectively to improve performance.
- The CPR Coach should be positioned next to the Defibrillator and in the direct line of sight of the Compressor.
- Because the CPR Coach must continually talk to give ongoing coaching, they must modulate their voice's tone and volume so that they do not disrupt other aspects of patient care.
- The CPR Coach should respect the Team Leader's role and not be perceived as trying to take over leadership. They should keep the Team Leader informed, share their understanding with the Team Leader, and ask for verification of key tasks and decisions.

Calculating CCF

Healthcare providers can calculate CCF mechanically by using a feedback device or manually by using 2 timers. One timer measures the total code time from code start until code stop or the return of spontaneous circulation, and a second timer measures the total chest compression time. To measure chest compression time, the second timer is started each time compressions begin or resume and is stopped during each pause in compressions. The chest compression time is then divided by the total code time to equal CCF:

CCF = actual chest compression time/total code time

Prebriefing

Effective briefing before a learning event, known as *prebriefing*, helps establish a safe environment for learning.

Educators can build a sense of psychological safety by prebriefing to let students know that mistakes are expected and serve as sources of learning and that interpersonal risk-taking is encouraged. Effective prebriefing builds rapport between students and instructors and encourages feedback receptivity by clarifying performance targets and explicitly outlining aspects of performance feedback relevant for the session so that students know what to expect: timing, sources, purpose (training or assessment), for example.

- Prebriefing should establish a supportive learning environment where it is safe to make mistakes and learn from them.
- This includes highlighting key performance goals and performance expectations, emphasizing the importance of ongoing practice, actively preparing students for the feedback they will receive, and describing when and how the debriefing will occur.
- Set rules and realism for the simulation.
- The high-performance team should establish goals and then discuss if those goals were met in the structured debriefing afterward.

Feedback and Coaching

At times, you will need to help a student master a skill. This may require expertise in communication and educational creativity. The fundamental principle of AHA courses is that students who are not able to master the required skills during the course can practice until they do. Instructors should be committed to finding and using the proper techniques that will be effective for a particular student. Adult learning principles coupled with debriefing techniques usually make for an effective combination. Here are some suggestions:

- Review the objectives for a particular scenario or skills station with the student.
- Give positive feedback when desired actions are observed; ask open-ended questions when nonpreferred actions are observed to determine the student's thought process.
- Use the same scenario repeatedly if necessary until the student accomplishes the objectives.

Debriefing

Debriefing is an organized, evidence-based, student-focused process that takes place in a nonthreatening environment. It is a method of assisting students in thinking about what they did, when they did it, why and how they did it, and how they can improve.

In an effective debriefing session, instructors ask questions and encourage students to analyze their own performance rather than offer only the instructor's perspective. Because this approach is focused on what the student thinks and does rather than on the instructor's viewpoint, students are more likely to remember and apply the lessons in their practice.

Feedback vs Debriefing

Simple feedback is typically geared toward correcting student actions the instructor has observed—an approach that can sometimes have the unintended consequence of fixing one mistake only to create others. Effective debriefing, on the other hand, focuses more on understanding why students acted a certain way, which allows correction of their thinking. Students typically do things for a reason that makes sense to them. Good debriefing helps students review their own performance and achieve a deeper understanding.

Although debriefing takes longer than simply giving feedback, reframing students' understanding will make the lesson more applicable to real life and will have a more lasting impact on future performance.

Effective Debriefing Characteristics

Effective debriefings must be fit for the purpose and focus on how to achieve performance standards. Specifically, instructors should attend to the established debriefing processes, tailor debriefings to context, use debriefing scripts to promote debriefing effectiveness, and view training as an opportunity to model debriefing practice and to prepare students for the process of a debriefing after actual clinical events.

Students need performance data to improve; these data should be included in debriefings whenever possible. Quantitative data provided during resuscitation education should come from several sources, including instructors, CPR devices, and data from simulators. Some data may be available in real time; other data, during debriefings.

Feedback and debriefing should be part of a larger curriculum design and should not occur in isolation. These powerful educational interventions are integral elements to overarching curriculum design considerations.

The characteristics of an effective debriefing session include

- Active participation
- Student discussion
- Self-analysis
- Application
- Thorough processing of information

With effective debriefing, students should

- Analyze and evaluate what happened
- Recognize how tools can help them manage situations
- Develop the habit of self-critique

We recommend using structured and supported debriefing, a learner-centered debriefing model that focuses on what the student knows and thinks. This approach draws on evidence-based findings from behavioral science to focus on critical thinking and encourage students to analyze their motivations and performance. It is an efficient and organized process to help students think about what they did—why, how, and when they did it—and how they can improve.

Structured and supported debriefing follows a simple 3-step format to achieve a comprehensive and effective debriefing:

- *Gather* information about the events.
- *Analyze* the information by using an accurate record.
- *Summarize* the attainment of objectives for future improvement.

Structured elements include the 3 specific phases described in Table 2, while supported elements include both interpersonal support and the use of protocols, algorithms, and best evidence. Be sure to allow enough time to conduct a debriefing session after each case scenario.

Table 2. Structured and Supported Debriefing Process

Phase	Goal	Actions
Gather	Ask what happened during the case, to develop a shared mental model of the events. Listen to students to understand what they think and how they feel about the simulation.	• Request a narrative from the Team Leader. • Request clarifying or supplementary information from the high-performance team.
Analyze	Facilitate students' reflection on and analysis of their actions.	• Review an accurate record of events. • Report observations (both correct and incorrect steps). • Assist students in thoroughly reflecting on and examining their performance during the simulation as well as in reflecting on their perceptions during the debriefing. • Direct and redirect students during the debriefing to ensure continuous focus on session objectives.
Summarize	Facilitate identification and review of the lessons learned that can be taken into actual practice.	• Summarize comments or statements from students. • Have students identify positive aspects of their high-performance team or individual behaviors. • Have students identify areas of their high-performance team or individual behaviors that require change or correction.

You should view yourself as a facilitator whose goals are to enhance learning during the training session and encourage students to critique themselves and reflect on future clinical encounters. This promotes continued self-improvement and will have a long-lasting effect well beyond any individual course.

A good facilitator effectively uses the key skills of listening, genuine inquiry, and open-ended questions to determine how the student understood the situation and what he or she was thinking. Correcting a particular action will have an impact on only a single behavior; correcting an approach will affect the student's actions in a variety of situations.

Appropriate pauses and silence can give students the time they need to formulate their thoughts. Demonstrating the usefulness of protocols and algorithms is also part of an effective facilitation.

Structured and supported debriefing can help facilitate learning the skills and techniques needed for clinical practice. It is also important that you model and encourage good debriefing techniques because debriefing of actual resuscitation events can be a useful strategy to help healthcare providers improve future performance in clinical practice.

Contextual Learning

Another core concept for resuscitation training is to use training experiences that apply to students' real-world scope of practice.

- Consider that different students find relevance in different things and tailor the learning experience for the types of students, their settings, and the resources available in their environment.
- When simulating resuscitation, acknowledge that manikin fidelity is not enough and use manikin features that matter. These features should engage students and be relevant to the learning objectives.
- Enhance realism for team training by ensuring that team composition, roles, and contexts are right for your student groups.
- Don't be afraid to stress your students (to a certain extent). The right amount of stress can enhance experiential learning by maximizing student engagement.

Testing for Course Completion

The AHA requires successful completion of skills tests, as well as an exam in instructor-led courses or successful completion of the online portion of HeartCode, for a student to receive a provider course completion card.

The prompt and accurate delivery of provider skills and knowledge is critically important for patient survival. Accurate, objective, and uniform testing reinforces these lifesaving skills and knowledge and is critical for the consistent delivery of content by all instructors.

All AHA Instructors are expected to maintain high standards of performance for all skills tests, as discussed in the following sections.

Skills Testing

During skills testing, students must demonstrate competency in all skills without any assistance, hints, or prompting from the instructor.

Instructors of the appropriate discipline will evaluate each student for his or her didactic knowledge and proficiency in all core psychomotor skills of the course. No AHA course completion card is issued without the required skills testing by either an AHA Instructor for that discipline or an AHA-approved computerized manikin in an AHA eLearning course.

Students in advanced life support courses are not required by the AHA to have a current BLS Provider card, but they are expected to demonstrate proficiency in BLS skills. Training Centers do have the option to require a current BLS Provider card, but requiring the card does not mean that BLS content and testing may be omitted from advanced courses.

Skills Testing of Blended-Learning Students

Instructors may need to conduct skills practice and testing during the hands-on session of a blended-learning course. The lesson plans in Part 6 will help facilitate these sessions. The skills testing portion of the hands-on session should be conducted the same as in an instructor-led course. Some skills tests may require that additional students be present while the tests are being conducted (refer to Part 4 for further details).

Exam

The exam measures the mastery of cognitive knowledge in ECC instructor-led healthcare courses. Each student must score at least 84% on the exam to meet course completion requirements.

The AHA has adopted an open-resource policy for exams administered through an eLearning course or in a classroom-based course. Open resource means that students may use resources as a reference while completing the exam. Resources could include the provider manual, either in printed form or as an eBook on personal devices, any notes the student took during the provider course, the 2020 Handbook of ECC for Healthcare Providers, the AHA Guidelines for CPR and ECC, posters, etc. Open resource does not mean open discussion with other students or the instructor. Students may not interact with each other during the exam.

In the welcome letter you send to students with their course materials, emphasize the importance of bringing their books to class to use during the exam. Students using the eBook version should download the manual to their device's eReader app and bring it with them in case there is no Internet connection.

Exams are administered online, though there may be an occasional need to administer a paper exam. More information about exams can be found on the Instructor Network.

If you use a paper exam, grade the exam, and answer any questions as soon as the student returns it. Students who score less than 84% will need to take a second exam or receive verbal remediation to confirm knowledge and understanding. If you give a student a second exam, review the first exam with the student, allowing them time to study the questions they got wrong. If you provide verbal remediation, ask the student to verbally answer the questions that he or she answered incorrectly, and document on the answer sheet whether the student correctly answered each question. You must document on the answer sheet that the remediation was successful, and that the student achieved a passing score.

If a student has difficulty reading or understanding the written questions, you may read the exam to the student. You must read the exam as written and in a manner that does not indicate the correct answer. You may verbally translate the exam if needed.

ECC blended-learning healthcare courses have a cognitive assessment incorporated into the online portion, so an exam does not need to be given to students when they attend the classroom portion.

Exam Security

Exam security is of the utmost importance:

- Ensure that all exams are kept secure and not copied or distributed outside the classroom.
- Exams are copyrighted; therefore, Training Centers or instructors may not alter them in any way or post them to any learning management systems such as Internet or intranet sites. This includes precourse self-assessments.*
- When a paper exam must be used, always print the most current version from the online exam platform for the course you are teaching.
- Each paper exam should be accounted for and returned to the instructor at the end of the testing period.

*Exams are translated into multiple languages. If a translated exam is needed for a course you are teaching, have your Training Center Coordinator contact ECC Customer Support to find out if the needed translation is available.

Remediation

Provider Course Student Remediation

At times, you will have to provide remediation to a student who is unable to perform satisfactorily in portions of the course. This is often resource-intensive and may require considerable expertise in communication and educational creativity.

The fundamental principle is that every student who is not able to master the required skills during the course is still able to benefit from remediation. The instructor should be committed to finding and using the proper techniques that will be effective for a student. Adult learning principles coupled with debriefing techniques usually make for an effective combination. Here are some suggestions:

- Review the objectives for a scenario or skills station with the student.
- Give positive feedback when desired actions are observed; ask open-ended questions when nonpreferred actions are observed to determine the student's thought process.
- Use the same scenario repeatedly if necessary until the student accomplishes the objectives.

Consider using another instructor to provide remediation because that instructor might be able to offer an alternative approach that will be helpful for the student.

At the time of the course, remediation for some students might not be successful within certain sections of the course (or exam or skills tests). When this happens, the student may arrange for a separate remediation session. A student must meet all learning objectives to the satisfaction of the Course Director or Lead Instructor before receiving a course completion card.

Students must complete all remediation sessions, including exams, skills tests, and skills stations, within 30 days after the last day of the original course. The remediation date will be listed as the issue date on the course completion card.

If a student does not successfully complete all course requirements within 30 days, the course is considered incomplete and a course completion card will not be issued.

Remediation Concepts for Instructors

Remediation is a learning process in which the instructor provides additional opportunities for the student to master the required skills of the course.

Informal remediation occurs throughout the course and is part of the learning process. When a student is having difficulty mastering a skill, he or she can be placed last in line for performing skills for practice and/or testing. This gives the student additional time to observe and learn from other students.

Formal remediation occurs after a student has been formally tested in a skills or core case testing station and has been unable to demonstrate mastery. Have the student work one-on-one with an instructor during breaks, lunchtime, or at the end of the day to assess areas for improvement in performing a skill. Then, encourage the student to practice and, when ready, to indicate when he or she wishes to be tested.

It is important to communicate the need for formal remediation in a private, sensitive, and objective debriefing immediately after the testing has taken place by using the scenario critical action objectives as a guide.

- Every student, with rare exceptions, should be able to benefit from remediation.
- Commit to providing remediation for students who have difficulties learning the skills and principles in the course the first time through.
- Instructor styles of facilitating and student styles of learning may not match; therefore, a change of instructor may be necessary.
- Don't assume that poor performance is associated with a lack of knowledge. There may be other factors (eg, personal or work-related issues) that are influencing the student's performance.
- If a student is still having difficulty after receiving remediation, you may need to examine the student's style of learning and make adjustments.
- The role of the instructor is to facilitate learning. Always be respectful, courteous, positive, professional, and diplomatic when providing remediation to a student.

Additional materials to assist in remediation will be provided in a later section of the manual.

Steps to Successful Remediation

You may find these steps helpful when providing remediation:

- Review the critical action steps that the student did not perform satisfactorily.
- Using open-ended questions (debriefing tool), assess the student's thought process, and correct it if necessary.
- Identify whether other factors might have affected the student's performance (eg, performance anxiety).
- Use the same or a similar scenario for retesting the student (eg, if the initial scenario was a respiratory case, use a respiratory case again for the retest).
- Use other students who need remediation or other instructors to help form a high-performance team to manage the case scenario.
- If performance anxiety or an instructor-student personality clash is a factor, ask another instructor to conduct the remediation.

Instructors should make every effort to correct knowledge and skills deficits during the course. Doing so can help minimize the chances that students will require formal remediation at the end of the course.

After the Course

Program Evaluation

Ongoing evaluation and improvement of AHA materials and instructors are important to the AHA. Each student should have an opportunity to evaluate the class. As an instructor, it is your responsibility to provide that opportunity. There are several options for how a course evaluation can be provided.

- Paper evaluation: A template for a written evaluation is available on the Instructor Network. Make enough copies so all your students can complete the evaluation at the end of the course and return it to you. Review the feedback, and then send the completed forms to your Training Center Coordinator.
- eCard survey (United States): If you are an instructor with a US Training Center and your Training Center is issuing eCards, your students will complete an online evaluation before they claim their course completion card. eCard surveys are another important way to gain valuable feedback from your students on their overall satisfaction of the course. eCard Reports are available on the Instructor Network.
- Online evaluation (international): If you are an instructor with an International Training Center, your students are encouraged to complete an evaluation online before they can claim their CPRverify™ course completion card (eCard); in addition, instructors can have students complete the paper evaluation located on CPRverify.

Issuing Provider Course Completion Cards

Each student who successfully completes the course requirements will be issued an AHA course completion card (eCard or printed). More information can be found on the Instructor Network.

No AHA course completion card is issued without hands-on manikin skills practice and testing by an AHA-approved computerized manikin as part of an AHA eLearning course or by an AHA Instructor for that discipline.

Continuing Education/Continuing Medical Education Credit for Courses

Most ECC online and blended courses offer continuing education (CE)/continuing medical education (CME) credit and are designed to meet CE criteria. The CE/CME certificate is automatically generated when students complete a course and claim their credit. This may not be the same as the certificate of completion.

Some classroom courses also offer credit for EMS professionals. The AHA is contracted to offer all EMS students CE hours through the Commission on Accreditation for Prehospital Continuing Education (CAPCE). Because there are contractual obligations to make CAPCE credit available to all EMS professionals completing a qualifying course, your Training Center and you, as an instructor, are required to collect and submit the information requested: first name, last name, and email address. The submission is done through the Instructor Network. Each student is then sent an email invitation to provide the additional needed information and claim his or her credit. While the information for all EMS students must be submitted, students are not obligated to accept or claim their certificates.

CAPCE accreditation does not represent that the content of a course conforms to any national, state, or local standard or best practice of any nature.

If you would like to offer CE credit to other professionals who attend your instructor-led courses, you will need to work with your Training Center or employer to apply for credit through the appropriate authorizing body.

Visit the Instructor Network to learn which courses offer CE/CME credit and to find more information and updates.

Provider Renewal

Renewal Timeline

The current recommended timeline for renewal of an AHA course completion card is every 2 years. Although there is insufficient evidence to determine the optimal method and timing of retaking a course, research on skills retention and training show the following:

- There is growing evidence that BLS knowledge and skills decay rapidly after initial training.
- Studies have demonstrated the deterioration of BLS skills in as little as months after initial training.
- Studies examining the effect of brief, more frequent training sessions demonstrated improvement in chest compression performance and shorter time to defibrillation.
- Studies also found that students reported improved confidence and willingness to perform CPR after additional or high-frequency training.

Given how fast BLS skills decay after training, and with the observed improvement in skills and confidence among students who train more frequently, students should be encouraged to periodically review their provider manuals and practice skills whenever possible. In addition, instructors and Training Centers may offer opportunities for students to practice and test their skills between course events.

Instructor Training

Recruiting and Mentoring Instructors

You may have students in your course who want to become AHA Instructors. The AHA encourages you, as a current AHA Instructor, to take a moment to pass along this information to all students who are interested in becoming an instructor after they successfully complete the provider course.

An AHA Instructor course teaches the methods needed to effectively teach others. The AHA requires that instructors be at least 18 years of age to attend an AHA Instructor course.

Instructor Candidate Selection

The ideal instructor candidate

- Is motivated to teach
- Is motivated to facilitate learning
- Is motivated to ensure that students acquire the skills necessary for successful course completion
- Views student assessment as a way to improve individual knowledge and skills

Instructor Course Prerequisites

Prospective participants in an AHA Instructor course must

- Have current provider status in the discipline they wish to teach
- Have completed an Instructor Candidate Application (obtained from the Training Center Coordinator)

Receiving an Instructor Card

Your instructor card for your discipline is issued by your primary Training Center. This may not be the same Training Center where you took your training or monitoring.

All instructor cards are valid for 2 years.

If you are a new instructor:

- You must be monitored teaching your first course within 6 months after completing the classroom portion of your training. A current Training Faculty member for your discipline must monitor you while you teach an initial provider course or an update or renewal course. It is your responsibility to schedule this monitoring, working with the Training Faculty member who conducted your course or with the Training Center Coordinator of your Training Center.
- You will receive your instructor card from your Primary Training Center once you have successfully completed all monitoring requirements. The expiration date will be 2 years from the month you completed all requirements, including monitoring.
- You must register on the Instructor Network with your Primary Training Center so that you receive your instructor ID number. This number is placed on the back of your card, so you need it before your card can be issued. Any questions about receiving your instructor card should be directed to your Training Center Coordinator.

Instructor Renewal Criteria: BLS

Your instructor status must be renewed by a Training Faculty member. You can renew your BLS instructor status by meeting all of the following criteria or by successfully completing all requirements for a new instructor.

- Maintain current provider status. You can do this by maintaining a current provider card or by demonstrating exceptional provider skills to a Training Faculty member and by successfully completing the provider exam.

- If you choose the demonstration route, successful completion must be documented on the Instructor/Training Faculty Renewal Checklist. A new provider card may be issued at the discretion of the Training Center or if you request one, but it is not required by the AHA.
- Earn 4 credits during each 2 years of your instructor recognition by doing any combination of the following:
  - Teach an instructor-led BLS or Heartsaver® class. Each class counts as 1 credit.
  - Conduct the hands-on skills session for a blended-learning course. Each day of HeartCode BLS hands-on sessions or Heartsaver hands-on sessions counts as 1 credit.
  - Conduct BLS and AED skills testing during a Pediatric Advanced Life Support (PALS); Pediatric Emergency Assessment, Recognition, and Stabilization (PEARS®); or Advanced Cardiovascular Life Support (ACLS) class. One credit is awarded per class.
  - Facilitate a Family & Friends® class. Each class counts as 1 credit.
- Attend updates as required within the previous 2 years. Updates may address new course content or methodology and review Training Center, regional, and national ECC information.
- Be monitored while teaching before instructor status expiration. The first monitoring after the Instructor Essentials Course does not satisfy this requirement.

Special Exceptions to Teaching Requirements

The requirement for instructors to teach a minimum of 4 courses in 2 years to renew instructor status may be waived or extended under special circumstances. These circumstances include, but are not limited to, the following:

- Call to active military duty (for an instructor who is in the military reserve or National Guard). Monitoring during duty may be waived if Military Training Network Faculty members are not available
- Illness or injury that has caused the instructor to take a leave from employment or teaching duties
- A limited number of courses offered in an area because of lack of audience or delay of course materials

The Training Center Coordinator, in consultation with the assigned Training Faculty, may decide to waive the teaching requirements for the discipline in question. Consideration should be given to the amount of time an instructor is away from normal employment, the length of delay in release of materials, and the number of courses taught in relation to the number of teaching opportunities. Documentation supporting the decision must be maintained in the instructor's file. All other requirements for renewal must be met as stated previously.

Preparing for the Course

Course Overview

Course Goal

The goal of the BLS Course is to train participants to save the lives of victims in cardiac arrest through high-quality CPR. The AHA designed the BLS Course to teach healthcare professionals how to perform high-quality CPR individually or as part of a team. BLS skills are applicable to any healthcare setting. BLS students will learn rescue techniques for adults, children, and infants.

Learning Objectives

At the end of the BLS Course, students will be able to

- Describe the importance of high-quality CPR and its impact on survival
- Describe all the steps of the Chain of Survival
- Apply the BLS concepts of the Chain of Survival
- Recognize when someone needs CPR
- Perform high-quality CPR for an adult, a child, and an infant
- Describe the importance of early use of an AED
- Demonstrate the appropriate use of an AED
- Provide effective ventilation by using a barrier device
- Describe the importance of teams in multirescuer resuscitation
- Perform as an effective team member during multirescuer CPR
- Describe how to relieve foreign-body airway obstruction for an adult, a child, and an infant

Educational Design

The AHA's BLS Course is designed for healthcare providers caring for patients both in and out of the hospital setting. Three different course formats are available to accommodate the learning needs of individual students and offer flexibility for instructors. All 3 course formats include the same learning objectives and result in the same course completion card. A list of available formats is below.

- Instructor-led training: This option is led by an instructor in a classroom setting. Instructors deliver courses designed to include both the cognitive portion of training and the psychomotor component of thorough skills practice and testing.
- Blended learning: Blended learning uses online technology not only to supplement but also to transform and improve the learning process. Successful blended learning can reach students with varying learning styles and in different environments. It is a combination of eLearning, in which a student completes part of the course in a self-directed manner, and a hands-on session with an instructor or a HeartCode-compatible manikin.

- Resuscitation Quality Improvement® (RQI®): A unique ECC program designed specifically for training actively employed healthcare providers in clinical environments. Unlike the traditional instructor-led and blended courses, the RQI program is a maintenance-of-competence platform designed for site-specific adoption.

Benefits of Blended Learning

The online component of the blended-learning experience benefits both students and instructors. Online learning accommodates many different learning styles. For example, some students prefer learning in a self-directed environment as opposed to a group setting. Also, online learning is time efficient for the following reasons:

- Students have the flexibility to take the online instruction whenever their schedules permit. Time spent at a Training Center or other facility for supervised practice and testing is reduced.
- Instructors have more time to focus on students' learning needs, such as answering questions, coaching, and skills development.
- Testing of core concepts is completed online, so students do not have to wait for other students to finish taking the exam, and instructors have more time to focus on students' learning needs.

Preparing to Teach HeartCode BLS

To be prepared to teach HeartCode BLS, the blended-learning program for BLS, we recommend that instructors take the online component of the course. This will help instructors understand what students learn there as well as answer questions students may have about the online course. As with instructor-led courses, all online courses are developed by using educational principles and best practices. Course materials are presented in a way that helps students learn and retain the information. Students are required to complete all online course activities, which are designed to teach and test core concepts. The online instruction is also designed to help students transfer and apply their knowledge to skills performance.

Instructors should review all course materials, including the instructor manual, skills testing checklists, critical skills descriptions, and skills sections of the course video. Because some students may require more in-depth information, instructors may want to review the high-performance teams and CCF sections in the course video as well.

Understanding HeartCode BLS

The online component of HeartCode BLS uses a variety of learning assets—such as dramatizations, animations, self-directed learning, and interactive activities—to teach students the knowledge and skills of BLS. After completing the online portion, students will complete a hands-on skills session either with a HeartCode-compatible manikin or by attending an instructor-led session that focuses on meaningful skills practice, debriefing, team scenarios, discussions of local protocols, and skills testing.

Validation of Online Course Certificates

When a student has completed the online portion of any AHA course, a skills practice and testing session must be completed with an AHA Instructor or an approved HeartCode-compatible manikin.

As a BLS Instructor, you may be asked to do a skills practice and testing session for HeartCode BLS or any of the Heartsaver online courses. You can confirm that the certificate a student brings you is valid.

 To validate a student's online completion certificate, go to **www.elearning.heart.org/verify_certificate**.

Course Audience

Who Can Take the Course

This course is designed for healthcare providers and trained first responders who provide care to patients in a wide variety of settings or by those in a healthcare training program.

Course Flexibility

The AHA allows instructors to tailor the BLS Course to meet audience-specific needs. Consider these examples:

- If you are teaching this course to staff at a children's hospital, you might want to include extra practice time on infant and child manikins.
- You may choose to adapt situations to the specific location.
- You may eliminate "phone 9-1-1" for students who are EMS professionals and other emergency responders.

Any changes to the course are in addition to the basic course contents as outlined in this manual and will add to the length of the course. Instructors may not delete course lessons or course components. Any additions or alterations to the course must be specifically identified as non-AHA material. Please refer to the section titled Non-AHA Content in this instructor manual for further detail.

Who Can Teach the Course

AHA courses must be taught by AHA Instructors who have current instructor status in their specific discipline. An AHA Instructor in the appropriate discipline must also perform the formal assessment or testing of students.

Lead Instructor

If more than 1 instructor is teaching in a BLS Course, a lead instructor needs to be designated. The lead instructor will oversee the communication among all instructors before and during the course. The lead instructor will also be responsible for issuing and ensuring that students receive course completion cards from the instructor's Training Center and that all course paperwork (eg, roster, skills testing checklists, course evaluations) is supplied for the training.

The following guidelines apply to lead instructors for provider courses:

- Each BLS Course must have a lead instructor physically on-site throughout the course.
- The lead instructor can also fill the role of instructor in the course.
- The lead instructor is responsible for course logistics and quality assurance.
- The lead instructor is assigned by the Training Center Coordinator.

Instructor-to-Student Ratio

The course size for the BLS Course is flexible. The course is designed for a ratio of 3 students to 1 manikin, with no more than 2 manikins to 1 instructor (6 students to 2 manikins to 1 instructor). With this ratio, 1 instructor observes 2 students during video-led manikin practice (practice while watching). The video for the course is designed to allow the practice-while-watching sections to be repeated as many times as needed.

Experienced instructors may monitor as many as 3 manikin stations at a time while the students practice. This would change the ratio to 9 students to 3 manikins to 1 instructor.

For optimal practice time during the course, each student should have his or her own manikin, if possible. However, using a 1:1 student-to-manikin ratio will not decrease overall class time. One instructor cannot adequately monitor more than 3 manikin stations during a single practice-while-watching video segment.

For skills evaluation, use a 1:1 instructor-to-student ratio.

Course Planning and Support Materials

Sample Precourse Letter to Students (Classroom Course)

The letter below is a sample you may modify and send to students attending the BLS Course.

(Date)

Dear BLS Course Student:

Welcome to the BLS Course. Enclosed are the agenda and your copy of the *BLS Provider Manual* to help you prepare for the program and the exam. Please bring your *BLS Provider Manual* to class; you will be able to refer to it during class and the exam. If you are using the eBook version, make sure your device is fully charged and download the manual to your device's eReader app in case there is no internet connection. Review both the agenda and the manual before coming to class so that you learn more and are more comfortable with the course.

The class is scheduled for

Date: _____

Time: _____

Location: _____

Please wear loose, comfortable clothing. You will be practicing skills that require working on your hands and knees, bending, standing, and lifting. If you have physical conditions that might prevent you from participating in the course, please tell one of the instructors when you arrive for class. The instructor will work to accommodate your needs within the stated course completion requirements. In the event that you are ill, please notify your instructor to reschedule your training.

We look forward to welcoming you on (day and date of class). If you have any questions about the course, please call (name) at (telephone number).

Sincerely,

(Name), Lead Instructor

Sample Precourse Letter to Students (HeartCode BLS)

The letter below is a sample you may modify and send to students completing HeartCode BLS.

(Date)

Dear BLS Course Student:

Welcome to the HeartCode® BLS Course. This course has 2 components: an online portion and an instructor-led classroom portion. You must complete the online portion first.

You can access the online portion of the course by using this unique URL: [student's license URL].

Important: You must print the certificate of completion at the end of the online portion. You will need to give this to your instructor when you attend the classroom portion. It is necessary to show that you completed the online portion. If you do not have your certificate of completion, you will not be able to complete the skills practice and testing of the course.

The classroom portion is scheduled for

Date: _____

Time: _____

Location: _____

Please wear loose, comfortable clothing. You will be practicing skills that require working on your hands and knees, bending, standing, and lifting. If you have physical conditions that might prevent you from participating in the course, please tell one of the instructors when you arrive for class. The instructor will work to accommodate your needs within the stated course completion requirements. In the event that you are ill, please notify your instructor to reschedule your training.

We look forward to welcoming you on (day and date of class). If you have any questions about the course, please call (name) at (telephone number).

Sincerely,

(Name), Lead Instructor

Room Requirements

When selecting a location for a BLS Course, make sure the room has

- Good acoustics
- A clean and well-maintained environment
- Bright lighting that can be adjusted for video presentations
- An instructor-controlled video player and a monitor or screen large enough to be viewed by all the students
- A chair for each student
- Ideally, a firm surface with adequate padding/protection for skills practice (eg, carpeted floors, sturdy table top, hospital bed, padded mats)
- A table for completing the exam

Sample Floor Plan

Figure 2 shows a sample floor plan. Arrange the room so that all students can see the video screen and instructors can monitor student groups during practice.

Figure 2. Sample floor plan.

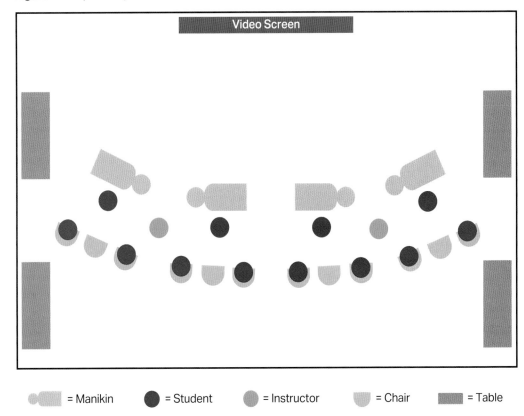

| | = Manikin | ● = Student | ● = Instructor | = Chair | = Table |

Core Curriculum

Each AHA course must follow the guidelines and core curriculum in the most current editions of the *BLS Provider Manual* and *BLS Instructor Manual*. Current editions of AHA course materials must serve as the primary training resources during the course.

Equipment List

Equipment required for each class held is listed in the table below. All equipment used must be in proper working order and good repair.

Course Materials

- **Course roster:** 1 per class
- **Course agenda:** 1 per instructor, 1 per student (if requested)
- **Lesson plans:** 1 per instructor
- **Course video:** 1 per class

Checklists and Exams

- **Skills testing checklists:** 1 per student
- **Exam version 1:** Paper copies as needed for backup for online exam (for classroom-based students)
- **Exam version 2:** Enough copies for remediation, if needed
- **Blank exam answer sheet:** 2 paper answer sheets per student as needed (for classroom-based students)
- **Exam answer key:** 1 for each exam version
- **Course evaluation:** 1 per student (for classroom-based students)
- **Pencil or pen:** 1 per student

Reference Material

- *BLS Instructor Manual*: 1 per instructor
- *BLS Provider Manual*: 1 per instructor, 1 per student

Equipment

- **AED trainer with adult and pediatric pads:** 1 per student group*
- **Manikins (adult/child, infant) (child manikin is optional):** 1 per student group*
- **Pocket mask:** 1 per student
- **Disposable mouthpiece:** 1 per student
- **Bag-mask device (appropriate sizes for each manikin used):** 1 per student
- **Stopwatches:** 2 per student
- **Video player and monitor or screen large enough for all students to view:** 1 per class
- **Manikin cleaning supplies (eg, alcohol pads):** 1 set per class

*Student group: 1 per group of 3 students if 3:1 student-to-manikin ratio, except during the High-Performance Teams Activity.

Part 3

Teaching the Course

Instructor Teaching Materials

Teaching Varied BLS Providers

The BLS Course is equipped to provide instruction to healthcare providers caring for patients both in and out of the hospital. The course's ability to serve both of these audiences is supported in the instructor-led (classroom) course and HeartCode BLS by both instructor and student materials.

Instructor-Led Training

The lessons featured on the video in the instructor-led BLS Course are based on real-world scenarios that show skills being demonstrated in settings for each type of BLS provider: in-facility provider or prehospital provider. To adapt to your classroom audience, as an instructor you have the option to choose between in-facility and prehospital lessons as you navigate through the video during the course.

Blended Learning

Students participating in HeartCode BLS experience the same tailoring to their needs by self-identifying as in-facility provider or prehospital provider. On the basis of their response, students navigate through the appropriate content of the online portion of the course. They view the same real-world scenarios featured in the instructor-led BLS video to prepare for skills practice and testing in the classroom.

The instructor manual, lesson plans, provider manual, and testing are designed to support both the instructor-led training and blended-learning formats of the course. Part 2: Preparing for the Course and Part 4: Testing will explain more about using each of these materials.

Understanding Icons

The icons used in the lesson plans, in this manual, and in the BLS Course videos are there to remind you to take certain actions during the course. The lesson plans and videos contain the following icons:

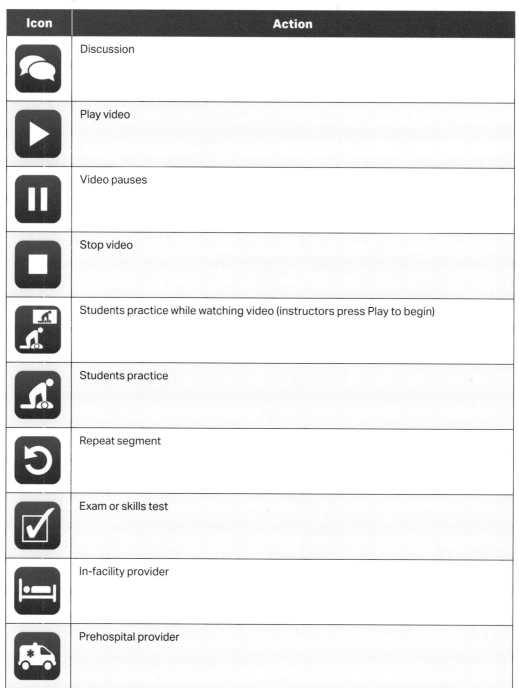

Icon	Action
	Discussion
	Play video
	Video pauses
	Stop video
	Students practice while watching video (instructors press Play to begin)
	Students practice
	Repeat segment
	Exam or skills test
	In-facility provider
	Prehospital provider

Understanding Lesson Plans

All AHA ECC instructor manuals include lesson plans (Figure 3). The purposes of lesson plans are to

- Help instructors facilitate ECC courses
- Ensure consistency from course to course
- Keep instructors focused on the main objectives for each lesson
- Explain the instructor's responsibilities during the course

Figure 3. Sample lesson plan.

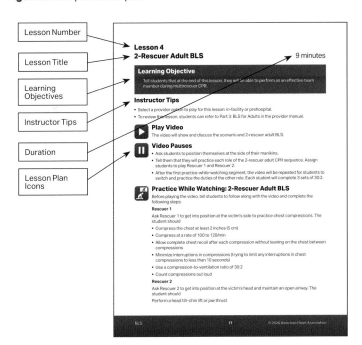

Using Lesson Plans

Use lesson plans before the course, during the course, and during skills practice.

Before the course:

Review the lesson plans to understand

- Objectives for each lesson
- Your role for each lesson
- Resources that you need for each lesson

Make notes of things you want to remember or add.

During the course:

- Follow each lesson plan as you conduct the course.
- Remind students what they will see in each video segment.
- Make sure you have all the resources, equipment, and supplies ready for each lesson.
- Help the students achieve the objectives identified for each lesson.

During practice before a skills test:

A student may have a question about a certain part of BLS. The lesson plans serve as the authoritative answer.

Teaching With a Video

The BLS Course and classroom portion of HeartCode BLS are video based. Many of the lessons in the BLS Course use the practice-while-watching format. This means that students practice skills as the video guides them. To make sure that course material is taught consistently and that students benefit from the latest scientific research, show all of the course's video lessons completely.

Practice While Watching

The practice-while-watching method is used to teach skills in the BLS Course. Practice while watching is an effective approach for building skills mastery.

Practice while watching aids the learning experience by organizing content into the following format:

- Tell students what they will learn
- Show them
- Allow them to practice
- Provide coaching
- Summarize what they learned

Instructors should use the video to demonstrate correct performance of skills. Allow students time to practice while following the video demonstration. Observe students' performance of the skills and provide corrective feedback. Finally, give students the option to practice without the video, if needed.

Using the Provider Manual

Each student must have the current *BLS Provider Manual* readily available for use before, during, and after the course.

Students will need to do the following with the provider manual:

- Read it before coming to class
- Bring it to class to use as a resource during the exam
- Refer to it after the course to maintain knowledge

The AHA designed this manual to correspond with the course video. The lesson plans tell you when to refer students to specific sections of the provider manual.

The provider manual is designed for individual use and is an integral part of the student's education. Students may reuse their manuals during renewals or updates until new science guidelines are published.

Students taking HeartCode BLS have access to the *BLS Provider Manual* and other reference materials within the eLearning course. They may access the reference materials for up to 2 years after the date of key activation. Students should be allowed to bring electronic devices into the classroom to access these electronic materials.

Course Outlines and Agendas

BLS Course Outline

Approximate course duration: 3 hours 40 minutes (for all required lessons); student-instructor ratio 6:1; student-manikin ratio 3:1; lesson times below are estimates and can vary from course to course

Lesson	Course event	Lesson plan actions and time estimate (in minutes)
Precourse	Precourse Preparation	
1	**Course Introduction**	5
2	**1-Rescuer Adult BLS** Part 1: Adult Chains of Survival Part 2: Scene Safety, Assessment, and Adult Compressions Part 3: Pocket Mask Part 4: 1-Rescuer Adult BLS	30
3	**AED and Bag-Mask Device** Part 1: AED Part 2: Bag-Mask Device	20
4	**2-Rescuer Adult BLS**	9
5	**Special Considerations** Part 1: Mouth-to-Mouth Breaths Part 2: Rescue Breathing Part 3: Breaths With an Advanced Airway Part 4: Opioid-Associated Life-Threatening Emergency Part 5: Maternal Cardiac Arrest	10
6	**High-Performance Teams** Part 1: Team Dynamics Part 2: High-Performance Teams Part 3: High-Performance Teams Activity (Optional)	26
6A (optional)	**Local Protocols Discussion**	20
7	**Child BLS** Part 1: Pediatric Chains of Survival Part 2: Child BLS Part 3: 2-Rescuer Child CPR	10

(continued)

Lesson	Course event	Lesson plan actions and time estimate (in minutes)		
8	**Infant BLS** Part 1: Infant BLS Part 2: Infant Compressions Part 3: Bag-Mask Device for Infants Part 4: 2-Rescuer Infant CPR Part 5: AED for Infants and Children Less Than 8 Years of Age	▶ ⏸ 🖼 ↺ 🖼 ☑ 20		
9	**Relief of Choking** Part 1: Adult and Child Choking Part 2: Infant Choking	▶ 💬 ⏸ 🖼 ◻ 7		
10	**Conclusion**	💬 5		
11	**Skills Test** Part 1: Adult CPR and AED Skills Test Part 2: Infant CPR Skills Test	💬 ☑ 40		
12	**Exam**	💬 ☑ 25		
13	**Remediation** Part 1: Skills Testing Remediation Part 2: Exam Remediation	▶ ☑ 15		
Postcourse	**Immediately After the Course**			

BLS Renewal Course Outline

Approximate course duration: 3 hours (for all required lessons); student-instructor ratio 6:1; student-manikin ratio 3:1; lesson times below are estimates and can vary from course to course

Lesson	Course event	Lesson plan actions and time estimate (in minutes)
Precourse	Precourse Preparation	
1	**Course Introduction**	5
2	**Adult BLS** Part 1: Adult Chains of Survival Part 2: 1-Rescuer Adult BLS Part 3: AED Practice Part 4: Bag-Mask Device	22
3	**Special Considerations** Part 1: Mouth-to-Mouth Breaths Part 2: Rescue Breathing Part 3: Breaths With an Advanced Airway Part 4: Opioid-Associated Life-Threatening Emergency Part 5: Maternal Cardiac Arrest	10
4	**High-Performance Teams** Part 1: Team Dynamics Part 2: High-Performance Teams Part 3: High-Performance Teams Activity (Optional)	26
4A (optional)	**Local Protocols Discussion**	20
5	**Child BLS** Part 1: Pediatric Chains of Survival Part 2: 2-Rescuer Child CPR Part 3: Adult CPR and AED Skills Test (Optional)	9
6	**Infant BLS** Part 1: Infant Compressions Part 2: 2-Rescuer Infant CPR Part 3: AED for Infants and Children Less Than 8 Years of Age Part 4: Infant CPR Skills Test (Optional)	18
7	**Relief of Choking** Part 1: Adult and Child Choking Part 2: Infant Choking	7

(continued)

Lesson	Course event	Lesson plan actions and time estimate (in minutes)
8	**Conclusion**	5
9	**Skills Test** Part 1: Adult CPR and AED Skills Test Part 2: Infant CPR Skills Test	40
10	**Exam**	25
11	**Remediation** Part 1: Skills Testing Remediation Part 2: Exam Remediation	15
Postcourse	**Immediately After the Course**	

HeartCode® BLS Outline

Approximate course duration: 2 hours (for all required lessons); student-instructor ratio 6:1; student-manikin ratio 3:1; lesson times below are estimates and can vary from course to course

Lesson	Course event	Lesson plan actions and time estimate (in minutes)
Precourse	Precourse Preparation	
1	**Course Introduction**	5
2	**Adult BLS** Part 1: Scene Safety, Assessment, and Adult Compressions Part 2: Pocket Mask Part 3: 1-Rescuer Adult BLS Part 4: Bag-Mask Device Part 5: 2-Rescuer Adult BLS	27
3	**AED for Adults, Children, and Infants** Part 1: AED Review Part 2: AED	10
4	**Special Considerations: Rescue Breathing**	3
5 (optional)	**High-Performance Teams Activity**	17
5A (optional)	**Local Protocols Discussion**	20
6	**2-Rescuer Child CPR**	7
7	**Infant BLS** Part 1: Infant Compressions Part 2: Bag-Mask Device for Infants Part 3: 2-Rescuer Infant CPR	15
8	**Relief of Choking** Part 1: Adult and Child Choking Part 2: Infant Choking	8

(continued)

Lesson	Course event	Lesson plan actions and time estimate (in minutes)
9	Conclusion	2
10	**Skills Test** Part 1: Adult CPR and AED Skills Test Part 2: Infant CPR Skills Test	40
11	Remediation*	
Postcourse	**Immediately After the Course**	

*Remediation time will vary depending on need and number of students.

Sample BLS Course Agenda With Optional Lessons

12 students, 2 BLS Instructors; student-instructor ratio 6:1; student-manikin ratio 3:1;
total time: approximately 4 hours and 15 minutes (with breaks)

Time	Lesson
8:00-8:05	**Lesson 1: Course Introduction**
8:05-8:35	**Lesson 2: 1-Rescuer Adult BLS** Part 1: Adult Chains of Survival Part 2: Scene Safety, Assessment, and Adult Compressions Part 3: Pocket Mask Part 4: 1-Rescuer Adult BLS
8:35-8:55	**Lesson 3: AED and Bag-Mask Device** Part 1: AED Part 2: Bag-Mask Device
8:55-9:04	**Lesson 4: 2-Rescuer Adult BLS**
9:04-9:14	**Lesson 5: Special Considerations** Part 1: Mouth-to-Mouth Breaths Part 2: Rescue Breathing Part 3: Breaths With an Advanced Airway Part 4: Opioid-Associated Life-Threatening Emergency Part 5: Maternal Cardiac Arrest
9:14-9:40	**Lesson 6: High-Performance Teams** Part 1: Team Dynamics Part 2: High-Performance Teams Part 3: High-Performance Teams Activity (Optional)
9:40-10:00	**Lesson 6A: Local Protocols Discussion (Optional)**
10:00-10:10	**Break**
10:10-10:20	**Lesson 7: Child BLS** Part 1: Pediatric Chains of Survival Part 2: Child BLS Part 3: 2-Rescuer Child CPR
10:20-10:40	**Lesson 8: Infant BLS** Part 1: Infant BLS Part 2: Infant Compressions Part 3: Bag-Mask Device for Infants Part 4: 2-Rescuer Infant CPR Part 5: AED for Infants and Children Less Than 8 Years of Age
10:40-10:47	**Lesson 9: Relief of Choking** Part 1: Adult and Child Choking Part 2: Infant Choking
10:47-10:52	**Lesson 10: Conclusion**
10:52-11:32	**Lesson 11: Skills Test** Part 1: Adult CPR and AED Skills Test Part 2: Infant CPR Skills Test

(continued)

Time	Lesson
11:32-11:57	**Lesson 12: Exam**
11:57-12:12	**Lesson 13: Remediation** Part 1: Skills Testing Remediation Part 2: Exam Remediation

Sample BLS Renewal Course Agenda Without Optional Lessons

6 students, 1 BLS Instructor; student-instructor ratio 6:1; student-manikin ratio 3:1;
total time: approximately 3 hours (with breaks)

Time	Lesson
8:00-8:05	**Lesson 1: Course Introduction**
8:05-8:27	**Lesson 2: Adult BLS** Part 1: Adult Chains of Survival Part 2: 1-Rescuer Adult BLS Part 3: AED Practice Part 4: Bag-Mask Device
8:27-8:37	**Lesson 3: Special Considerations** Part 1: Mouth-to-Mouth Breaths Part 2: Rescue Breathing Part 3: Breaths With an Advanced Airway Part 4: Opioid-Associated Life-Threatening Emergency Part 5: Maternal Cardiac Arrest
8:37-8:46	**Lesson 4: High-Performance Teams** Part 1: Team Dynamics Part 2: High-Performance Teams
8:46-8:56	**Break**
8:56-9:05	**Lesson 5: Child BLS** Part 1: Pediatric Chains of Survival Part 2: 2-Rescuer Child CPR
9:05-9:23	**Lesson 6: Infant BLS** Part 1: Infant Compressions Part 2: 2-Rescuer Infant CPR Part 3: AED for Infants and Children Less Than 8 Years of Age
9:23-9:30	**Lesson 7: Relief of Choking** Part 1: Adult and Child Choking Part 2: Infant Choking
9:30-9:35	**Lesson 8: Conclusion**
9:35-10:15	**Lesson 9: Skills Test** Part 1: Adult CPR and AED Skills Test Part 2: Infant CPR Skills Test
10:15-10:40	**Lesson 10: Exam**
10:40-10:55	**Lesson 11: Remediation** Part 1: Skills Testing Remediation Part 2: Exam Remediation

Sample HeartCode® BLS Agenda With Optional Lessons

12 students, 2 BLS Instructors; student-instructor ratio 6:1; student-manikin ratio 3:1;
total time: approximately 2 hours 35 minutes

Time	Lesson
8:00-8:05	**Lesson 1: Course Introduction**
8:05-8:32	**Lesson 2: Adult BLS** Part 1: Scene Safety, Assessment, and Adult Compressions Part 2: Pocket Mask Part 3: 1-Rescuer Adult BLS Part 4: Bag-Mask Device Part 5: 2-Rescuer Adult BLS
8:32-8:42	**Lesson 3: AED for Adults, Children, and Infants** Part 1: AED Review Part 2: AED
8:42-8:45	**Lesson 4: Special Considerations: Rescue Breathing**
8:45-9:02	**Lesson 5: High-Performance Teams Activity (Optional)**
9:02-9:22	**Lesson 5A: Local Protocols Discussion (Optional)**
9:22-9:29	**Lesson 6: 2-Rescuer Child CPR**
9:29-9:44	**Lesson 7: Infant BLS** Part 1: Infant Compressions Part 2: Bag-Mask Device for Infants Part 3: 2-Rescuer Infant CPR
9:44-9:52	**Lesson 8: Relief of Choking** Part 1: Adult and Child Choking Part 2: Infant Choking
9:52-9:54	**Lesson 9: Conclusion**
9:54-10:34	**Lesson 10: Skills Test** Part 1: Adult CPR and AED Skills Test Part 2: Infant CPR Skills Test
	Lesson 11: Remediation*

*Remediation time will vary depending on need and number of students.

Sample HeartCode® BLS Agenda Without Optional Lessons

12 students, 2 BLS Instructors; student-instructor ratio 6:1; student-manikin ratio 3:1;
total time: approximately 2 hours

Time	Lesson
8:00-8:05	**Lesson 1: Course Introduction**
8:05-8:32	**Lesson 2: Adult BLS** Part 1: Scene Safety, Assessment, and Adult Compressions Part 2: Pocket Mask Part 3: 1-Rescuer Adult BLS Part 4: Bag-Mask Device Part 5: 2-Rescuer Adult BLS
8:32-8:42	**Lesson 3: AED for Adults, Children, and Infants** Part 1: AED Review Part 2: AED
8:42-8:45	**Lesson 4: Special Considerations: Rescue Breathing**
8:45-8:52	**Lesson 6: 2-Rescuer Child CPR**
8:52-9:07	**Lesson 7: Infant BLS** Part 1: Infant Compressions Part 2: Bag-Mask Device for Infants Part 3: 2-Rescuer Infant CPR
9:07-9:15	**Lesson 8: Relief of Choking** Part 1: Adult and Child Choking Part 2: Infant Choking
9:15-9:17	**Lesson 9: Conclusion**
9:17-9:57	**Lesson 10: Skills Test** Part 1: Adult CPR and AED Skills Test Part 2: Infant CPR Skills Test
	Lesson 11: Remediation*

*Remediation time will vary depending on need and number of students.

Testing

Testing for Course Completion

Course Completion Requirements

To receive a course completion card, students must complete all cognitive components of the course, either through the instructor-led course or HeartCode BLS. Students in the instructor-led course must also pass a cognitive exam with a passing score of at least 84%. In addition, students must pass all psychomotor skills assessments, including independent skills test showing proficiency as outlined on the Adult CPR and AED and Infant CPR Skills Testing Checklists. Skills tests will be completed with a feedback device to ensure requirements are met.

When to Give Tests

You will test students as outlined in the lesson plans.

Skills testing is performed during the hands-on skills session of HeartCode BLS or in the instructor-led course. It can be administered during the course or at the end, at the discretion of the instructor. Please refer to the lesson plans for when to administer skills testing.

The cognitive exam is administered at the conclusion of the BLS Course. HeartCode BLS has cognitive assessment incorporated throughout the online portion, so an exam does not need to be given to HeartCode students.

Skills Testing

As part of the emphasis on better teaching and learning, the AHA developed CPR skills tests to ensure that there is a uniform and objective approach for testing CPR skills.

The skills testing checklists help instructors evaluate each student's CPR skills. The AHA-approved HeartCode-compatible manikin is designed to align with the skills testing checklists. As a result of the course design and skills tests, the AHA expects that students in CPR classes will learn more effectively and instructors will work with students to achieve higher levels of CPR skills competency.

CPR competency is critical to victim survival. It is important that you use the skills testing checklists to evaluate each student's performance and to ensure consistent testing and learning across all AHA BLS courses. In addition, students must use a CPR feedback device during skills tests, allowing you to accurately monitor their compression rate, depth, and recoil as well as ventilation rate and volume. Your adherence to these testing procedures will enhance the CPR competency of your students.

You must keep a copy of completed skills testing checklists for students who are unsuccessful. For records retention, refer to the *Program Administration Manual*.

Using a Stopwatch

To achieve accuracy during the skills practice and testing, a stopwatch is used to measure the rate of compressions. Follow these rules when using a stopwatch:

- Start your stopwatch when the student first compresses the breastbone.
- Stop your stopwatch at the end of the 30th compression.
- Mark the step correct if the number of seconds is between 15 and 18 seconds.

Using the Skills Testing Checklists and Critical Skills Descriptors

Use the skills testing checklists to document the student's performance during the skills testing portion of the course. The skills testing checklist should be filled out while the student is performing the skills. Use the skills testing critical skills descriptors to determine if a student has demonstrated each step of the skill correctly.

If the student successfully completes a step, place a check (✓) in the box to the left of the step on the skills testing checklist.

If the student is unsuccessful, leave the box next to the step blank on the skills testing checklist. Circle the step under the critical skills descriptor that the student did not complete successfully.

If a student demonstrates each step of the skills test successfully, mark the student as passing that skills test on the skills testing checklist. If a student does not receive checks in all boxes, refer the student to the remediation lesson at the end of the course for further testing in that skill. Also, discuss with the student the areas that you circled on the critical skills descriptors and how to correctly perform each skill that was circled.

You should be very familiar with all the critical skills descriptors to be able to test BLS skills correctly.

Understanding the Adult CPR and AED Skills Testing Checklist

Assessment and Activation

The steps in this box do not have to be completed in a specific order; the student only needs to complete all of the steps before beginning compressions. In addition, the student must take no less than 5 seconds and no more than 10 seconds to check breathing and check a pulse (ideally these checks should be done at the same time).

Once the student shouts for help, the instructor should say, "Here's the barrier device. I am going to get the AED."

Adult Compressions

During this section, evaluate the student's ability to perform high-quality chest compressions. Feedback devices are required to objectively evaluate chest compressions, and high-fidelity manikins are recommended as the optimal feedback device. Compressions should be initiated within 10 seconds after recognizing cardiac arrest.

Hand Placement

Evaluate the student to ensure that hand placement is on the lower half of the breastbone (sternum) and that the heel of the hand is used. When the student uses 2 hands, the second hand is placed on top of or grasping the wrist of the first hand.

Rate

Compression rate should be evaluated by using a feedback device and a stopwatch. To achieve a rate of 100 to 120 compressions per minute, students should deliver 30 compressions in 15 to 18 seconds.

Depth and Recoil

Evaluating depth and recoil in the absence of a feedback device or a manikin is unreliable. To increase the validity and reliability of the test, you must use commercial feedback devices or manikins that have the capability to objectively evaluate depth and recoil. High-fidelity manikins, with lights or an electronic display that indicates correct depth and recoil, are highly recommended. Manikins with a depth indicator that makes a clicking sound when compressions are deep enough are acceptable.

Tip: To help students achieve adequate compression depth and to minimize fatigue, instruct them to perform chest compressions with their elbows locked and their shoulders over the victim.

Adult Breaths

Breaths should be given only with a barrier device, such as a pocket mask or face shield. The device used should be similar to what the students will be using in their workplace. If the type of device is unknown, instructors should provide students with the device they used in training. In some circumstances, a workplace may have only a bag-mask device available. In these instances, students may complete their skills test with a bag-mask device. Instructors should emphasize that in the clinical setting, a rescuer will not be able to deliver 2 breaths within 10 seconds when using a bag-mask device during 1-rescuer CPR.

Each Breath Given Over 1 Second

Students should open the victim's airway by using the head tilt–chin lift. Each student should deliver 2 breaths. Each breath should be given over 1 second while the student observes for chest rise.

Visible Chest Rise

Students should deliver just enough air for visible chest rise.

Tip: If students are having difficulty providing breaths, ensure that they have a proper seal and that the airway is open. You might need to help students with their hand placement on the pocket mask or bag-mask device so that they can get a proper seal.

Minimizing Interruptions

The pause from the end of the last compression in a cycle to the beginning of the first compression of the next cycle should be no more than 10 seconds. This can be challenging to achieve with a bag-mask device.

Adult Cycle 2

Students should deliver another set of 30 compressions and 2 breaths. Evaluate students with the same criteria as in Cycle 1.

Adult AED

The second rescuer (either another student or the instructor) may participate in the delivery of CPR or bring the AED.

The instructor or a second student can arrive with an AED and hand it to the first student. The second student or the instructor can take over compressions. If a second student is not available, the instructor can hand the student the AED and instruct the student to use the AED. The instructor can tell the student that another rescuer is providing chest compressions. It is important that students understand that the attachment of AED pads should not interrupt chest compressions.

The student should turn the AED on as required for his or her specific device; this may require the student to push the power button on the AED, or the AED may turn on automatically when the case is opened. Students should attach the AED pads to the manikin by following the pictures on the pads. Students should follow the prompts of the AED they are using. Instructors should be aware that some of the AED steps outlined on the skills testing checklist might not be completely applicable to all devices. Some AEDs require the patient to be cleared during the analysis and charging cycle, and some AEDs allow compressions to be continued while the device is charging. Instructors should encourage their students to contact the manufacturer of their particular device to understand the device's capabilities. Once the AED is ready to deliver a shock, the student should clear the patient both verbally and visually. Once everyone is clear, the student should press the shock button and then resume compressions immediately.

Note: An AED is not used in infant testing.

Resumes Compressions

The student being evaluated should begin compressions immediately after the shock is delivered or tell the instructor to begin compressions immediately after the shock is delivered. Evaluate the student's ability to begin compressions immediately after the shock delivery. Evaluate the student with the same criteria for compressions as in Cycle 1; if the student resumes compressions or directs the instructor to begin compressions immediately, stop the test.

Test Results

If the student successfully performs all of the skills, circle "Pass" on the student's skills testing checklist. If the student does not successfully perform all of the skills, circle "NR" for needs remediation. The instructor should retest (reevaluate) the student on the skills that were not performed correctly by using a new skills testing checklist. If remediation is needed, both the skills testing checklist that indicated the need for remediation and the new skills testing checklist indicating that the student passed should be stored with the course records. Provide your initials, your instructor ID, and the date in the box at the end of the checklist.

Basic Life Support
Adult CPR and AED
Skills Testing Checklist

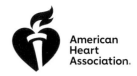
American Heart Association®

Student Name _____ Date of Test _____

Hospital Scenario: "You are working in a hospital or clinic, and you see a person who has suddenly collapsed in the hallway. You check that the scene is safe and then approach the patient. Demonstrate what you would do next."

Prehospital Scenario: "You arrive on the scene for a suspected cardiac arrest. No bystander CPR has been provided. You approach the scene and ensure that it is safe. Demonstrate what you would do next."

Assessment and Activation

☐ Checks responsiveness   ☐ Shouts for help/Activates emergency response system/Sends for AED

☐ Checks breathing   ☐ Checks pulse

Once student shouts for help, instructor says, "Here's the barrier device. I am going to get the AED."

Cycle 1 of CPR (30:2) **CPR feedback devices are required for accuracy*

Adult Compressions

☐ Performs high-quality compressions*:

• Hand placement on lower half of sternum

• 30 compressions in no less than 15 and no more than 18 seconds

• Compresses at least 2 inches (5 cm)

• Complete recoil after each compression

Adult Breaths

☐ Gives 2 breaths with a barrier device:

• Each breath given over 1 second

• Visible chest rise with each breath

• Resumes compressions in less than 10 seconds

Cycle 2 of CPR (repeats steps in Cycle 1) *Only check box if step is successfully performed*

☐ Compressions   ☐ Breaths   ☐ Resumes compressions in less than 10 seconds

---

Rescuer 2 says, "Here is the AED. I'll take over compressions, and you use the AED."

AED (follows prompts of AED)

☐ Powers on AED   ☐ Correctly attaches pads   ☐ Clears for analysis

☐ Clears to safely deliver a shock   ☐ Safely delivers a shock

---

Resumes Compressions

☐ Ensures compressions are resumed immediately after shock delivery

• Student directs instructor to resume compressions *or*

• Second student resumes compressions

STOP TEST

Instructor Notes

• Place a check in the box next to each step the student completes successfully.

• If the student does not complete all steps successfully (as indicated by at least 1 blank check box), the student must receive remediation. Make a note here of which skills require remediation (refer to instructor manual for information about remediation).

Test Results	Circle **PASS** or **NR** to indicate pass or needs remediation:	**PASS**	**NR**

Instructor Initials _____   Instructor Number _____   Date _____

Basic Life Support
Adult CPR and AED
Skills Testing Critical Skills Descriptors

1. **Assesses victim and activates emergency response system (this *must* precede starting compressions) within 30 seconds. After determining that the scene is safe:**
   - Checks for responsiveness by tapping and shouting
   - Shouts for help/directs someone to call for help *and* get AED/defibrillator
   - Checks for no breathing or no normal breathing (only gasping)
     - Scans from the head to the chest for a minimum of 5 seconds and no more than 10 seconds
   - Checks carotid pulse
     - Can be done simultaneously with check for breathing
     - Checks for a minimum of 5 seconds and no more than 10 seconds

2. **Performs high-quality chest compressions (initiates compressions immediately after recognition of cardiac arrest)**
   - Correct hand placement
     - Lower half of sternum
     - 2-handed (second hand on top of the first or grasping the wrist of the first hand)
   - Compression rate of 100 to 120/min
     - Delivers 30 compressions in 15 to 18 seconds
   - Compression depth and recoil—at least 2 inches (5 cm) and avoid compressing more than 2.4 inches (6 cm)
     - Use of a commercial feedback device or high-fidelity manikin is required
     - Complete chest recoil after each compression
   - Minimizes interruptions in compressions
     - Delivers 2 breaths so less than 10 seconds elapses between last compression of one cycle and first compression of next cycle
     - Compressions resumed immediately after shock/no shock indicated

3. **Provides 2 breaths by using a barrier device**
   - Opens airway adequately
     - Uses a head tilt–chin lift maneuver or jaw thrust
   - Delivers each breath over 1 second
   - Delivers breaths that produce visible chest rise
   - Avoids excessive ventilation
   - Resumes chest compressions in less than 10 seconds

4. **Performs same steps for compressions and breaths for Cycle 2**

5. **AED use**
   - Powers on AED
     - Turns AED on by pushing button or lifting lid as soon as it arrives
   - Correctly attaches pads
     - Places proper-sized (adult) pads for victim's age in correct location
   - Clears for analysis
     - Clears rescuers from victim for AED to analyze rhythm (pushes analyze button if required by device)
     - Communicates clearly to all other rescuers to stop touching victim
   - Clears to safely deliver shock
     - Communicates clearly to all other rescuers to stop touching victim
   - Safely delivers a shock
     - Resumes chest compressions immediately after shock delivery
     - Does not turn off AED during CPR

6. **Resumes compressions**
   - Ensures that high-quality chest compressions are resumed immediately after shock delivery
     - Performs same steps for compressions

Understanding the Infant CPR Skills Testing Checklist

Assessment and Activation

The steps in this box do not have to be completed in a specific order; the student only needs to complete all of the steps before beginning compressions. In addition, the student must take no less than 5 seconds and no more than 10 seconds to check breathing and check a pulse (ideally these checks should be done at the same time).

Once the student shouts for help, the instructor should say, "Here's the barrier device."

Infant Compressions

During this section, evaluate the student's ability to perform high-quality chest compressions. Feedback devices are required to objectively evaluate chest compressions, and high-fidelity manikins are recommended as the optimal feedback device. Compressions should be initiated within 10 seconds after recognizing cardiac arrest.

Finger Placement, Cycles 1 and 2 (1-Rescuer CPR)

Evaluate the student to ensure that finger or thumb placement is in the center of the chest and 2 fingers or 2 thumbs are placed just below the nipple line.

Finger Placement, Cycle 3 (2-Rescuer CPR)

Evaluate the student's 2 thumb–encircling hands technique for infant compressions during 2-rescuer CPR. Ensure that the student's 2 thumbs are placed on the lower half of the breastbone, just below the nipple line.

Rate, Cycles 1 and 2 (1-Rescuer CPR)

Compression rate should be evaluated by using a feedback device and a stopwatch. To achieve a rate of 100 to 120 compressions per minute, students should deliver 30 compressions in 15 to 18 seconds.

Rate, Cycle 3 (2-Rescuer CPR)

Compression rate should be evaluated by using a feedback device and a stopwatch. To achieve a rate of 100 to 120 compressions per minute, students should deliver 15 compressions in 7 to 9 seconds.

Depth and Recoil

Evaluating depth and recoil in the absence of a feedback device or a manikin is unreliable. To increase the validity and reliability of your testing experience, you must use commercial feedback devices that have the capability to objectively evaluate depth and recoil. High-fidelity manikins, with lights or an electronic display that indicates correct depth and recoil, are highly recommended. Manikins with a depth indicator that makes a clicking sound when compressions are deep enough are acceptable. If the student cannot achieve the recommended depth, you can tell the student that it may be reasonable to use the heel of 1 hand.

Infant Breaths

Breaths should be given only with a barrier device, such as a pocket mask or face shield. The device used should be similar to what the students would be using in their workplace. If the type of device is unknown, instructors should provide students with the device they used in training. In some circumstances, a workplace may have only a bag-mask device available. In these instances, students may complete their skills test with a bag-mask device. Instructors should emphasize that in the clinical setting, a rescuer will not be able to deliver 2 breaths within 10 seconds when using a bag-mask device during 1-rescuer CPR.

Breaths, Cycle 4 (2-Rescuer CPR)

Breaths should be given with a bag-mask device.

Each Breath Given Over 1 Second

Students should open the victim's airway by using the head tilt–chin lift. Each student should deliver 2 breaths. Each breath should be given over 1 second while the student observes for chest rise.

Visible Chest Rise

Students should deliver just enough air for visible chest rise.

Tip: If students are having difficulty providing breaths, ensure they have a proper seal and that the airway is open. You might need to help students with their hand placement on the pocket mask or bag-mask device so that they can get a proper seal.

Minimizing Interruptions

The pause from the end of the last compression in a cycle to the beginning of the first compression of the next cycle should be no more than 10 seconds. This can be challenging to achieve with a bag-mask device.

Infant Cycle 2

Students should deliver another 30 compressions and 2 breaths. Evaluate students with the same criteria as in Cycle 1.

Infant Cycle 3

The student being evaluated continues compressions while the second rescuer (either another student or the instructor) gets in position to provide breaths with a bag-mask device. The student being evaluated should provide compressions with the 2 thumb–encircling hands technique, with the 2 thumbs placed on the lower half of the breastbone, just below the nipple line. The test will end once the student has paused after 15 compressions so that the second rescuer can deliver 2 breaths.

Note: The students will switch roles at the end of this cycle, before Cycle 4.

Infant Cycle 4

The second student can continue compressions while the student being evaluated gets in position to provide breaths with a bag-mask device. After a cycle of 15 compressions, the student being evaluated should provide 2 breaths by using a bag-mask device. Each breath should be delivered over 1 second. Each breath should result in visible chest rise. There should be no more than a 10-second pause in compressions for the breaths to be delivered.

Test Results

If the student successfully performs all of the skills, circle "Pass" on the student's skills testing checklist. If the student does not successfully perform all of the skills, circle "NR" for needs remediation. The instructor should retest (reevaluate) the student on the skills that were not performed correctly by using a new skills testing checklist. If remediation is needed, both the skills testing checklist that indicated the need for remediation and the new skills testing checklist indicating that the student passed should be stored with the course records. Provide your initials, your instructor ID, and the date in the box at the end of the checklist.

Basic Life Support
Infant CPR
Skills Testing Checklist (1 of 2)

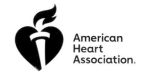

American Heart Association.

Student Name _____   Date of Test _____

Hospital Scenario: "You are working in a hospital or clinic when a woman runs through the door, carrying an infant. She shouts, 'Help me! My baby's not breathing.' You have gloves and a pocket mask. You send your coworker to activate the emergency response system and to get the emergency equipment."

Prehospital Scenario: "You arrive on the scene for an infant who is not breathing. No bystander CPR has been provided. You approach the scene and ensure that it is safe. Demonstrate what you would do next."

Assessment and Activation

☐ Checks responsiveness   ☐ Shouts for help/Activates emergency response system

☐ Checks breathing   ☐ Checks pulse

Once student shouts for help, instructor says, "Here's the barrier device."

Cycle 1 of CPR (30:2)   ***CPR feedback devices are required for accuracy***

Infant Compressions

☐ Performs high-quality compressions*:

• Placement of 2 fingers or 2 thumbs in the center of the chest, just below the nipple line

• 30 compressions in no less than 15 and no more than 18 seconds

• Compresses at least one third the depth of the chest, approximately 1½ inches (4 cm)

• Complete recoil after each compression

Infant Breaths

☐ Gives 2 breaths with a barrier device:

• Each breath given over 1 second

• Visible chest rise with each breath

• Resumes compressions in less than 10 seconds

Cycle 2 of CPR (repeats steps in Cycle 1)   ***Only check box if step is successfully performed***

☐ Compressions   ☐ Breaths   ☐ Resumes compressions in less than 10 seconds

---

Rescuer 2 arrives with bag-mask device and begins ventilation while Rescuer 1 continues compressions with 2 thumb–encircling hands technique.

Cycle 3 of CPR

Rescuer 1: Infant Compressions

☐ Performs high-quality compressions*:

• 15 compressions with 2 thumb–encircling hands technique

• 15 compressions in no less than 7 and no more than 9 seconds

• Compresses at least one third the depth of the chest, approximately 1½ inches (4 cm)

• Complete recoil after each compression

Rescuer 2: Infant Breaths

This rescuer is not evaluated.

(continued)

Basic Life Support
Infant CPR
Skills Testing Checklist (2 of 2)

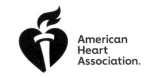
American
Heart
Association.

Student Name _____   Date of Test _____

(continued)

Cycle 4 of CPR

Rescuer 2: Infant Compressions

This rescuer is not evaluated.

Rescuer 1: Infant Breaths

☐ Gives 2 breaths with a bag-mask device:

- Each breath given over 1 second
- Visible chest rise with each breath
- Resumes compressions in less than 10 seconds

STOP TEST

Instructor Notes

- Place a check in the box next to each step the student completes successfully.
- If the student does not complete all steps successfully (as indicated by at least 1 blank check box), the student must receive remediation. Make a note here of which skills require remediation (refer to instructor manual for information about remediation).

Test Results	Circle **PASS** or **NR** to indicate pass or needs remediation:	**PASS**	**NR**
Instructor Initials _____ Instructor Number _____ Date _____			

Basic Life Support
Infant CPR
Skills Testing Critical Skills Descriptors

1. **Assesses victim and activates emergency response system (this *must* precede starting compressions) within 30 seconds. After determining that the scene is safe:**
   - Checks for responsiveness by tapping and shouting
   - Shouts for help/directs someone to call for help *and* get emergency equipment
   - Checks for no breathing or no normal breathing (only gasping)
     - Scans from the head to the chest for a minimum of 5 seconds and no more than 10 seconds
   - Checks brachial pulse
     - Can be done simultaneously with check for breathing
     - Checks for a minimum of 5 seconds and no more than 10 seconds

2. **Performs high-quality chest compressions during 1-rescuer CPR (initiates compressions within 10 seconds after identifying cardiac arrest)**
   - Correct placement of hands/fingers in center of chest
     - 1 rescuer: 2 fingers or 2 thumbs just below the nipple line
     - *If the rescuer is unable to achieve the recommended depth, it may be reasonable to use the heel of one hand*
   - Compression rate of 100 to 120/min
     - Delivers 30 compressions in 15 to 18 seconds
   - Adequate depth for age
     - Infant: at least one third the depth of the chest (approximately 1½ inches [4 cm])
     - Use of a commercial feedback device or high-fidelity manikin is required
   - Complete chest recoil after each compression
   - Appropriate ratio for age and number of rescuers
     - 1 rescuer: 30 compressions to 2 breaths
   - Minimizes interruptions in compressions
     - Delivers 2 breaths so less than 10 seconds elapses between last compression of one cycle and first compression of next cycle

3. **Provides effective breaths with bag-mask device during 2-rescuer CPR**
   - Opens airway adequately
   - Delivers each breath over 1 second
   - Delivers breaths that produce visible chest rise
   - Avoids excessive ventilation
   - Resumes chest compressions in less than 10 seconds

4. **Switches compression technique at appropriate interval as prompted by the instructor (for purposes of this evaluation). Switch should take no more than 5 seconds.**

5. **Performs high-quality chest compressions during 2-rescuer CPR**
   - Correct placement of hands/fingers in center of chest
     - 2 rescuers: 2 thumb–encircling hands just below the nipple line
   - Compression rate of 100 to 120/min
     - Delivers 15 compressions in 7 to 9 seconds
   - Adequate depth for age
     - Infant: at least one third the depth of the chest (approximately 1½ inches [4 cm])
   - Complete chest recoil after each compression
   - Appropriate ratio for age and number of rescuers
     - 2 rescuers: 15 compressions to 2 breaths
   - Minimizes interruptions in compressions
   - Delivers 2 breaths so less than 10 seconds elapses between last compression of one cycle and first compression of next cycle

Retesting Students

If time permits during skills testing, you may retest a student 1 additional time if the student did not pass. If a student does not pass a skills test after the second attempt, work with the student during the remediation lesson at the end of the course and retest at that time. All additional retesting is done at the end of the course during the remediation lesson. In every retesting case, test the student in the entire skill. In some cases, you may defer retesting to a later time after the course. For example, if remediation is not successful, you might develop a plan of improvement and schedule retesting once the student completes the plan. If a student needs substantial additional remediation, you may recommend that the student repeat a BLS course.

BLS Lesson Plans

Precourse Preparation

Instructor Tips

- Prepare for your role as a BLS Instructor well. Review all course materials and anticipate questions or challenges that may arise during the course. The time you invest in this part of your preparation is important to the overall success of every student.

- Refer to Part 3: Teaching the Course for further instructions on using lesson plans.

30 to 60 Days Before Class

- Determine course specifics, such as

  - Your students' professions (in-facility or prehospital providers) and how they'll use the skills taught in this course

  - The number of students

  - Any special equipment needed for the course

- Reserve the equipment you need for the course. Refer to Part 2: Preparing for the Course for a complete equipment list.

- Schedule a room that meets BLS Course requirements. Refer to Part 2: Preparing for the Course for details.

- Schedule additional instructors, if needed, depending on your class size.

At Least 3 Weeks Before Class

- Send participating students the precourse letter, course agenda, and student materials.

- Confirm any additional scheduled instructors.

- Research local protocols and encourage students to know them before coming to class. This will help you answer students' questions during the course. Refer to optional Lesson 6A: Local Protocols Discussion in the BLS Lesson Plans for more details and examples.

Day Before Class

- Confirm room reservations and ensure that all required equipment is available.
- Set up the room and make sure that all technology and equipment work. You can do this the day of class if the room is not accessible the day before.
- Locate the nearest AED in the building and confirm the emergency response number.
- Coordinate all roles and responsibilities with any additional instructors to ensure efficiency and timing, per the course agenda.
- Ensure that all course paperwork is in order.
- If you will be using the Full Code Pro app for the high-performance teams activity, download the app to an iOS smartphone or tablet. Review the app before class to become familiar with the functionality.

Day of Class

Arrive at the course location in plenty of time to complete the following:

- Make sure that all equipment works and has been cleaned according to manufacturer instructions.
- Have the video ready to play before students arrive.
- Distribute supplies to the students or set up supplies for students to collect when they arrive, with clear instructions on what they need.
- Greet students as they arrive to put them at ease, and direct them where to go.
- Make sure students complete the course roster as they arrive.

Lesson 1
Course Introduction

5 minutes

Instructor Tips

- Be familiar with the learning objectives and BLS Course content. It's critical that you know what you want to communicate, why it's important, and what you want to happen as a result.

- Prebrief the students. Explain that this is a safe space for learning and that mistakes are expected as part of the learning process. Students can practice skill repetition with your feedback to improve their performance. Remind students that they must demonstrate mastery of key resuscitation skills to successfully complete the course.

- Tailor the learning experience to students' real-world scope of practice, if possible. Consider the types of students, their settings, and the resources that are available to them. Structure team training so that scenarios, team composition, and roles are relevant.

- Think about how you'll manage breaks during the course. Consider using the time to establish rapport, get feedback, and answer questions students might feel too embarrassed to ask in front of everyone.

Discussion

- Introduce yourself and any additional instructors.

- Invite students to introduce themselves.

- Explain that the course is interactive. Discuss your role, video-based learning, the provider manual, the scenarios, practice while watching, and skills tests and the exam.

  - Refer to Part 3: Teaching the Course for detailed information about practice while watching.

- Ask students to speak to an instructor if they anticipate difficulties due to medical concerns, such as knee or back problems. Refer to Part 1: General Concepts for more about students with special needs.

- Explain the layout of the building, including bathrooms and emergency exits.

- Tell students the location of the nearest AED and the emergency response number.

- Describe the course agenda, including when you'll have breaks and when the class will end.

- Remind students that at the end of the BLS Course, they will be able to

  - Describe the importance of high-quality CPR and its impact on survival

  - Describe all of the steps of the Chain of Survival

  - Apply the BLS concepts of the Chain of Survival

  - Recognize the signs of someone needing CPR

  - Perform high-quality CPR for an adult, a child, and an infant

  - Describe the importance of using an AED as soon as possible

  - Demonstrate the appropriate use of an AED

  - Provide effective ventilation by using a barrier device

- Describe the importance of teams in multirescuer resuscitation attempts
- Perform as an effective team member during multirescuer CPR
- Describe the techniques for relief of foreign-body airway obstruction for an adult, a child, and an infant

- For further detail on the video and scenarios to be shown during the course, refer to the BLS Course Outline in Part 3: Teaching the Course.
- Remind students that to complete the course, they must
  - Pass the Adult CPR and AED Skills Test
  - Pass the Infant CPR Skills Test
  - Score at least 84% on the exam

Lesson 2
1-Rescuer Adult BLS

30 minutes

Part 1: Adult Chains of Survival

Part 2: Scene Safety, Assessment, and Adult Compressions (Practice While Watching)

Part 3: Pocket Mask (Practice While Watching)

Part 4: 1-Rescuer Adult BLS (Practice While Watching)

Learning Objectives

Tell students that at the end of this lesson, they will be able to

- Describe the importance of high-quality CPR and its impact on survival
- Describe all of the steps of the Chain of Survival
- Apply the BLS concepts of the Chain of Survival
- Recognize the signs of someone needing CPR
- Perform high-quality CPR for an adult

Instructor Tips

- Remind students that they will be practicing while watching a video segment so that they are prepared to get into place quickly to practice.
- When students are practicing, focus your feedback on what you *do* want rather than what you *don't* want. Always state feedback in a positive tone.
- Tell students to have their provider manuals accessible during the course.
- When concluding a practice-while-watching session, ask students if they are ready to move to the next skill or if they would like to repeat practice while watching.
- Learn how to assemble and operate the equipment that students will use in class. Be prepared to help them with it as needed and troubleshoot any problems.
- Select a provider option to play for this lesson: in-facility or prehospital.
- To review this lesson, students can refer to Part 3: BLS for Adults in the provider manual.

Play Video

The video will show the scenario and discuss the adult Chains of Survival, scene safety, assessment, and adult compressions.

Video Pauses

- Ask students to position themselves at the side of their manikins.
- Tell them that they will practice being the first rescuer on the scene, checking for scene safety, and assessing the victim. In addition, they will practice adult compressions, completing 3 sets of 30 compressions.

Practice While Watching: Scene Safety, Assessment, and Adult Compressions

Scene Safety and Assessment

Before playing the video, tell students to follow along with the video and complete the actions for scene safety and assessment. Tell students the following:

- Verify that the scene is safe for you and the victim.
- Check for responsiveness. Tap the victim's shoulder and shout, "Are you OK?"
- If the victim is not responsive, shout for nearby help.
- Assess the victim for the presence of a pulse and normal breathing.
- Activate the emergency response system in your setting.
- Get the AED. If someone else is available, have that person get it.

You can also remind students that it's important to know where to find personal protective equipment in their work environment.

Adult Compressions

Before playing the video, tell students to follow along with the video and complete the steps for adult compressions. Tell students the following:

- Position yourself at the victim's side.
- Put the heel of one hand on the center of the victim's chest, on the lower half of the breastbone (sternum).
- Put the heel of your other hand on top of the first hand.
- Straighten your arms and position your shoulders directly over your hands.
- Give chest compressions:
  - Press down at least 2 inches (5 cm) with each compression. Make sure you push straight down on the victim's breastbone.
  - Deliver compressions at a rate of 100 to 120/min.
  - Allow complete chest recoil after each compression without leaning on the chest between compressions.
- Minimize interruptions in chest compressions (trying to limit any interruptions in chest compressions to less than 10 seconds).

Emphasize core concepts: Use correct hand placement, push hard and fast, allow complete chest recoil after each compression, and minimize pauses in compressions.

Play Video

The video will show and discuss pocket masks.

Video Pauses

- Ask students to position themselves at the side of their manikins.
- Tell them that they will practice using a pocket mask and complete 5 sets of 2 breaths.

Practice While Watching: Pocket Mask

Before playing the video, tell students to follow along with the video and complete the steps for using a pocket mask. Tell students the following:

- Position yourself at the victim's side.
- Place the pocket mask on the victim's face, using the bridge of the nose as a guide for correct position.
- Seal the pocket mask against the face:
  - Using your hand that is closer to the top of the victim's head, place the index finger and thumb along the edge of the mask that is on the nose.
  - Place the thumb of your other hand along the edge of the mask that is on the chin.
- Place the remaining fingers of your second hand along the bony margin of the jaw and lift the jaw. Perform a head tilt–chin lift to open the airway.
- While you lift the jaw, press firmly and completely around the outside edge of the mask to seal the pocket mask against the face.
- Deliver each breath over 1 second, enough to make the victim's chest rise.

Tell students to hold the mask firmly against the face. Emphasize visible chest rise.

Play Video

The video will show and discuss 1-rescuer adult BLS.

Video Pauses

- Ask students to position themselves at the side of their manikins.
- Tell them that they will practice the entire 1-rescuer adult BLS sequence and complete 3 sets of 30 compressions, with 2 breaths after each set of compressions.

Practice While Watching: 1-Rescuer Adult BLS

Before playing the video, tell students to follow along with the video. They will complete the steps for scene safety and assessment, adult compressions, and pocket mask. Refer to each skill in this lesson plan for detailed steps. Coach students to perform high-quality CPR and minimize pauses in compressions. The interval of time between breaths and compressions should be as short as possible.

Lesson 3
AED and Bag-Mask Device

20 minutes

Part 1: AED (Students Practice)

Part 2: Bag-Mask Device (Practice While Watching)

Learning Objectives

Tell students that at the end of this lesson, they will be able to

- Describe the importance of early use of an AED
- Demonstrate the appropriate use of an AED
- Provide effective ventilation by using a barrier device

Instructor Tips

- Select a provider option to play for this lesson: in-facility or prehospital.
- To review this lesson, students can refer to Part 4: Automated External Defibrillator for Adults and Children 8 Years of Age and Older and Part 3: BLS for Adults in the provider manual.

Play Video

The video will show and discuss the use of an AED and a bag-mask device, including AED special considerations, such as if the person

- Has a hairy chest
- Is immersed in water or has water covering the chest
- Has an implanted defibrillator or pacemaker
- Has a transdermal medication patch or other object on the surface of the skin where the AED pads need to be placed
- Is an infant or child less than 8 years of age
- Is a pregnant woman

Video Pauses: AED Review

During the pause, show students the AED trainer and

- Explain how to use the AED trainer; remind students that it will not deliver a real shock
- Emphasize following the AED prompts
- Direct students to have their AED trainers out and ready to use
- Tell students that they are now going to practice using the AED

Students Practice: AED

Provide the following instructions on how to use an AED. First show the steps while using your AED trainer, and then ask students to practice.

Instructions for Students

1. Open the carrying case. Power on the AED if needed.

   – Some devices will power on automatically when you open the lid or case.

   – Follow the AED prompts for the next steps.

2. Attach AED pads to the victim's bare chest.

   – Choose adult pads (not child pads or a child system) for victims 8 years of age and older.

   – Peel the backing from the AED pads.

   – Attach the adhesive AED pads to the victim's bare chest. Place one pad on the manikin's upper-right chest (directly below the collarbone). Place the other pad to the side of the left nipple, with the top edge of the pad a few inches below the armpit.

   – Attach the AED connecting cables to the AED box (some are preconnected).

3. Clear the manikin and analyze the rhythm.

   – If the AED prompts you, clear the victim during analysis. Be sure no one is touching the victim, not even the rescuer in charge of giving breaths.

   – Some AEDs will tell you to push a button to allow the AED to begin analyzing the heart rhythm; others will do that automatically. The AED may take a few seconds to analyze.

   – The AED then tells you if a shock is needed.

4. If the AED advises a shock, it will tell you to clear the victim.

   – Clear the victim before delivering the shock; be sure no one is touching the victim.

   – Loudly state a "clear the victim" message, such as "Everybody clear" or simply "Clear."

   – Look to be sure no one is in contact with the victim.

   – Press the shock button.

5. The shock will produce a sudden contraction of the victim's muscles.

6. If the AED prompts that no shock is advised, or after any shock is delivered, immediately resume CPR, starting with chest compressions.

Play Video

The video will show and discuss bag-mask devices.

Video Pauses

- Ask students to position themselves at the side of their manikins.

- Tell them that they will practice using the bag-mask device and complete 5 sets of 2 breaths.

Practice While Watching: Bag-Mask Device

Before playing the video, tell students to follow along with the video and complete the steps for using a bag-mask device. Tell students the following:

- Position yourself directly above the victim's head.
- Place the mask on the victim's face, using the bridge of the nose as a guide for correct position.
- Use the E-C clamp technique to hold the mask in place while you lift the jaw to hold the airway open.
  - Perform a head tilt–chin lift.
  - Place the mask on the face, with the narrow portion at the bridge of the nose.
  - Use the thumb and index finger of one hand to form a C on the side of the mask, pressing the edges of the mask to the face.
  - Use the remaining fingers to lift the angles of the jaw (3 fingers form an E), open the airway, and press the face to the mask.
- Squeeze the bag to give breaths (1 second each) while watching for chest rise. Deliver each breath over 1 second, whether or not you use supplemental oxygen.
  - Instructors: Make sure students give 2 breaths and watch for chest rise.

Lesson 4
2-Rescuer Adult BLS

9 minutes

Learning Objective

Tell students that at the end of this lesson, they will be able to perform as an effective team member during multirescuer CPR.

Instructor Tips

- Select a provider option to play for this lesson: in-facility or prehospital.
- To review this lesson, students can refer to Part 3: BLS for Adults in the provider manual.

Play Video

The video will show and discuss the scenario and 2-rescuer adult BLS.

Video Pauses

- Ask students to position themselves at the side of their manikins.
- Tell them that they will practice each role of the 2-rescuer adult CPR sequence. Assign students to play Rescuer 1 and Rescuer 2.
- After the first practice-while-watching segment, the video will be repeated for students to switch and practice the duties of the other role. Each student will complete 3 sets of 30:2.

Practice While Watching: 2-Rescuer Adult BLS

Before playing the video, tell students to follow along with the video and complete the following steps:

Rescuer 1

Ask Rescuer 1 to get into position at the victim's side to practice chest compressions. The student should

- Compress the chest at least 2 inches (5 cm)
- Compress at a rate of 100 to 120/min
- Allow complete chest recoil after each compression without leaning on the chest between compressions
- Minimize interruptions in compressions (trying to limit any interruptions in chest compressions to less than 10 seconds)
- Use a compression-to-ventilation ratio of 30:2
- Count compressions out loud

Rescuer 2

Ask Rescuer 2 to get into position at the victim's head and maintain an open airway. The student should

- Perform a head tilt–chin lift or jaw thrust

- Give breaths with a bag-mask device, watching for chest rise and avoiding excessive ventilation

Tell Rescuer 2 to encourage Rescuer 1 to perform compressions that are deep enough and fast enough and to allow complete chest recoil after each compression.

Observe students and provide positive and corrective feedback on their performance.

Repeat Segment

Ask students to switch roles and repeat the practice-while-watching segment.

Students Practice (Optional): 2-Rescuer Adult BLS With AED

- After students complete the 2-rescuer CPR sequence in the practice-while-watching segment, tell them to incorporate the AED into their full adult CPR sequence.
  - Follow the steps on the Adult CPR and AED Skills Testing Checklist for how to use the AED in a 2-rescuer CPR sequence.
- Observe students and provide positive and corrective feedback, while emphasizing
  - Arrival and activation of the AED
  - Correct placement of the AED pads
  - Following the AED prompts
- Make sure all students complete the practice session.

Lesson 5
Special Considerations

10 minutes

Part 1: Mouth-to-Mouth Breaths

Part 2: Rescue Breathing (Practice While Watching)

Part 3: Breaths With an Advanced Airway

Part 4: Opioid-Associated Life-Threatening Emergency

Part 5: Maternal Cardiac Arrest

Instructor Tips

- Select a provider option to play for this lesson: in-facility or prehospital.

- To review this lesson, students can refer to Part 8: Alternate Ventilation Techniques and Part 9: Opioid-Associated Life-Threatening Emergencies in the provider manual.

Play Video

The video will show and discuss mouth-to-mouth breaths and rescue breathing.

Video Pauses

- Ask students to position themselves at the side of their manikins.

- Tell them that they will practice rescue breathing on the manikin.

- You may ask students to practice rescue breathing on infant manikins instead of adult manikins. If selecting this option, go to Students Practice: Rescue Breathing (Infants and Children) instead of Practice While Watching: Rescue Breathing (Adults).

Practice While Watching: Rescue Breathing (Adults)

Before playing the video, tell students to follow along with the video and complete the steps for adult rescue breathing. Tell students the following:

- Give 1 breath every 6 seconds.

- Give each breath over 1 second, ensuring that each breath results in visible chest rise.

- Check the pulse about every 2 minutes.

Students Practice: Rescue Breathing (Infants and Children)

Discuss and then ask students to practice the following steps for providing rescue breathing for infants and children:

- Give 1 breath every 2 to 3 seconds (about 20 to 30 breaths per minute).

- Give each breath over 1 second.

- Each breath should result in visible chest rise.

- Check the pulse about every 2 minutes

Play Video

The video will show and discuss breaths with an advanced airway, opioid-associated life-threatening emergencies, and maternal cardiac arrest.

- Advanced airway
  - No pauses in compressions
  - Adults: 1 breath every 6 seconds
  - Children and infants: 1 breath every 2 to 3 seconds
- Opioid-associated life-threatening emergencies
  - In all instances of opioid-associated life-threating emergencies, activate emergency medical services
  - If the victim is breathing and has a pulse, monitor breathing and consider naloxone
  - If the victim is not breathing and has a pulse, provide rescue breathing and give naloxone
  - If the victim is not breathing and has no pulse, start CPR
- Maternal cardiac arrest
  - Compressions, ventilation, and AED use remain unchanged for a pregnant woman
  - Manual displacement of the rounded abdomen to mother's left side (lateral uterine displacement) should be done if enough rescuers are present to continue with CPR

Lesson 6
High-Performance Teams

26 minutes

Part 1: Team Dynamics

Part 2: High-Performance Teams

Part 3: High-Performance Teams Activity (Optional)

Learning Objective

Tell students that at the end of this lesson, they will be able to describe the importance of teams in multirescuer resuscitation.

Instructor Tips

- To engage students during discussion, ask open-ended questions that elicit students' own unique perspectives. This will help increase participation.

- When answering a question, make eye contact to acknowledge the student. Then, address the entire room. From time to time, direct your attention back to the student who asked the question.

- The Team Dynamics portion of this lesson focuses on the elements of effective team dynamics, including the roles everyone must play. The High-Performance Teams portion of the lesson focuses on the skills needed to achieve specific performance metrics, including a high CCF.

- CCF is the proportion of time that rescuers perform chest compressions during CPR. Shorter duration of interruptions in chest compressions is associated with a better outcome. A CCF of at least 60% increases the likelihood of return of spontaneous circulation, shock success, and survival to hospital discharge. With good teamwork, rescuers can often achieve 80% CCF or more. In a 10-minute scenario, total chest compression time must be about 8 minutes to achieve an 80% CCF.

- Explain that BLS providers are responsible for performing only the roles on a resuscitation team that are within their training and scope of practice. It is important, however, to understand all team roles to be an effective team member.

- Select a provider option to play for this lesson: in-facility or prehospital.

- To review this lesson, students can refer to Part 5: Team Dynamics in the provider manual.

 ## Play Video: Team Dynamics

The video will show and discuss good team dynamics; team roles, including Team Leader, Compressor, Airway, IV/IO/Medications, Monitor/Defibrillator/CPR Coach, and Timer/Recorder; and the following information about successful resuscitation teams:

- The roles of each member

  - Clear roles and responsibilities

  - Knowing your limitations

  - Constructive intervention (be tactful)

- What to communicate
  - Knowledge sharing and frequently asking for observations
  - Summarizing and reevaluating, which can help respond to the patient's changing condition
- How to communicate
  - Closed-loop communication
  - Confirm order
  - Call people by their names
  - Confirm intervention complete
  - Clear messages
  - Speak in a calm, confident manner
  - Mutual respect
  - Behave in a professional manner
  - Use a friendly, controlled voice
  - Avoid shouting or aggression
- Debriefing
  - Debrief together as a team
  - Debrief after a resuscitation attempt
  - Debriefing may improve team performance and patient outcomes after cardiac arrest
- CPR Coach
  - The CPR Coach supports performance of high-quality BLS skills, allowing the Team Leader to focus on other aspects of clinical care. Studies have shown that resuscitation teams with a CPR Coach perform higher-quality CPR with higher CCF and shorter pause durations compared with teams that don't use a CPR Coach. This role was briefly covered in the Team Dynamics portion of this lesson.
  - The CPR Coach focuses only on compressions and ventilation to ensure high-quality CPR. They help minimize the length of pauses during provider switches and defibrillation.
  - The CPR Coach should be positioned next to the Defibrillator and in the direct line of sight of the Compressor.
  - Because the CPR Coach must continually talk to give ongoing coaching, they must adjust their tone and volume so that they do not disrupt other aspects of patient care.
  - The CPR Coach should respect the Team Leader's role and not be perceived as trying to take over leadership. They should keep the Team Leader informed, share their understanding with the Team Leader, and ask for verification of key tasks and decisions.
  - Any healthcare professional can be a CPR Coach if they have a current BLS Provider card, understand the responsibilities of a CPR Coach, and demonstrate the ability to coach Compressors and Airway providers effectively to improve performance.

Video Resumes: High-Performance Teams

The video will show and discuss the following information about the skills needed to achieve specific high-performance team metrics like CCF by eliminating the pauses commonly seen in a resuscitation attempt. Some key concepts covered include

- Hovering hands over the chest when compressions are paused
- Advanced providers checking the pulse and precharging the defibrillator about 15 seconds before pausing compressions every 2 minutes
- Switching Compressors every 2 minutes or whenever a Compressor is fatigued, with the second Compressor coming in behind the first
- Using real-time feedback devices during CPR, or a metronome if a feedback device is not available

Play Video: High-Performance Teams Activity (Optional)

The video will show and discuss the high-performance teams activity.

Instructor Tips

- During this activity, watch the performance of multiple rescuers simultaneously. Take note of team performance that can be improved to inform topics of discussion during the debriefing. You will present one 10-minute scenario and follow with a 5-minute debriefing.
- While students practice, you will calculate the CCF.

How Do I Measure CCF?

Option 1: Use 2 stopwatches.

1. Start one stopwatch once you have given the scenario to the team. Let it run continuously to the 10-minute mark (total resuscitation time) as a reminder to stop the case.

2. Use a second stopwatch to measure total compression time during the scenario. Start the stopwatch each time a Compressor starts chest compressions. Pause the stopwatch when the Compressor stops or when chest compressions are interrupted. Do this for each set of compressions during the entire scenario. Don't reset the stopwatch during the scenario; allow the stopwatch to continue counting up. This will give you the cumulative time that chest compressions were being performed during the scenario.

3. Convert the time on the second stopwatch to seconds (eg, 8 minutes = 480 seconds).

4. Divide the total compression time in seconds by the total resuscitation time in seconds (ie, 10 minutes = 600 seconds).

5. This will give you the CCF. For example, if the time on the second stopwatch is 520 seconds, divide by 600 (total resuscitation time): 520/600=0.8667. Then, round to 2 places and convert to a percentage: 87%.

Option 2: Use the AHA's Full Code Pro app. This app is a free, easy-to-use, mobile application that allows rescuers to document critical interventions during CPR. You can use Full Code Pro during real resuscitation events or in practice scenarios. Go to **https://itunes.apple.com/us/app/full-code-pro/id589451064?mt=8** to download the app for iOS devices. A Full Code Pro Tutorial video is available on the AHA Instructor Network.

Option 3: Use a manikin that captures resuscitation data.

Video Pauses

- Divide students into groups for the scenario. Assign team roles. Explain that after you read the scenario, students will begin the high-performance teams activity, which will run for 10 minutes. You will evaluate the resuscitation, looking for high-quality CPR and ensuring that students enforce the principles of highly effective teams. Briefly remind students that you will be tracking CCF because limiting interruptions in chest compressions improves outcome.

- Begin CCF tracking as soon as the Compressor begins chest compressions during CPR.

Students Practice

Read this scenario to each team:

- "As part of a multirescuer emergency response team, you respond to a call about a 65-year-old woman who suddenly collapsed. Your team arrives within seconds after the incident, and you notice that a bystander is performing compression-only CPR."

- Coach students in teamwork throughout the activity. Monitor CPR performance to inform high-quality CPR coaching, including minimizing pauses in compressions during the use of the AED. Provide focused practice as needed.

- Pay particular attention to the Compressor's performance toward the end of each 2-minute rotation. Monitor for high-quality compressions of adequate rate and depth. Remind the Compressor to allow complete chest recoil after each compression without leaning on the chest between compressions.

Discussion: High-Performance Teams Activity Debriefing

- At the end of the scenario, debrief by asking team members what they thought went well and what could have been better.
  - Disclose the CCF and discuss any strategies for improvement.
  - Talk about whether the team maintained high-quality CPR.
  - Allow the team to lead the conversation; ask open-ended questions to facilitate discussion.

- Coach on improving communication with closed-loop communication principles:
  - The Team Leader gives a message, an order, or an assignment to a team member.
  - The team member gives a clear response and makes eye contact to confirm that they heard and understood the message.
  - The Team Leader listens for confirmation of task performance from the team member before assigning another task.

Lesson 6A
Local Protocols Discussion (Optional)

20 minutes

Instructor Tips

- Across the country, EMS systems develop treatment protocols based on local need, preference of administration, and medical direction. In some cases, these protocols differ from established national standards, so this course may occasionally direct providers to act in ways that are not consistent with their local protocols. The AHA does not want to conflict with established local protocols.

- When you lead this discussion, make sure you know what the local protocols are. If you are a member of the local EMS system, you should already be aware of local protocols, but if you are not, study them before the course so that you can have a meaningful discussion.

Although the AHA does not endorse a particular protocol or strategy, it does issue evidence-based guidelines, which are relevant and broadly applicable. These guidelines are developed by experts in the field, who use a rigorous, scientific process. This discussion is a chance for students to articulate and practice AHA skills within the context of their local protocols.

Discussion

Lead students through a discussion about high-performance teams and local protocols. Use these questions to help guide this discussion:

- Does your system currently use a high-performance team approach to resuscitation?

- How can you incorporate high-performance teamwork into your department's protocols?

- What are some potential challenges to incorporating high-performance teamwork into your protocols?

- What are some potential challenges to high-performance teamwork in terms of location, patients, or equipment?

- How does the local protocol compare and contrast with the AHA BLS Healthcare Provider Adult Cardiac Arrest Algorithm?

The following examples show some common differences between local protocols and what is taught in the course. Use these sections only if students ask questions about these examples.

What to say when local protocols for chest compressions differ from what the course teaches:

In the course, you learned to do 30 high-quality chest compressions and then 2 breaths. This could differ from your local protocol, which may have you do 90 seconds of continuous chest compressions or 200 chest compressions before beginning breaths, or a variation of these.

- Follow the local protocol.

- The important factors in this lesson are to perform the compressions at a rate of 100 to 120/min, at least 2 inches in depth, while allowing the chest to recoil completely after each compression.

- The next Compressor should be immediately ready to switch roles to minimize interruption in compressions.

Studies show that patients who receive chest compressions at a rate of 100 to 120/min and a CCF of greater than 80% have a much better chance of survival.

What to say when local protocols for AED use differ from what the course teaches:

In the course, you learned to use the AED immediately after it arrives. This could differ from your local protocol, which may have you use the AED only after you do 200 chest compressions (or 2 minutes of CPR) or a variation of this.

- Follow the local protocol.
- Continue high-quality chest compressions up to the point of allowing the AED to analyze.
- Immediately begin chest compressions after a shock is delivered or the AED states, "no shock advised."
- Keep in mind that as time to defibrillation increases, the chance of survival decreases.

The greatest chance of survival from cardiac arrest is found when a patient receives high-quality CPR and early defibrillation.

What to say when local protocols for role assignment differ from what the course teaches:

In the course, you learned about the different roles that prehospital providers may have (Compressor, Timer/Recorder, etc). This could differ from your workplace protocol, which assigns you a role based on your role on the fire engine, ambulance, or other team.

- Follow the local protocol.
- Know your potential assignments ahead of time to reduce confusion during a real event.
- Make sure that all roles and responsibilities are clear so that interruptions in chest compressions are minimized and teamwork is smooth and efficient.
- It is critical that high-performance teams practice in the same way that they will perform in real situations.
- Appoint a Team Leader who oversees the event, assesses the efficacy of efforts, and makes changes when resuscitation performance is less than adequate.
- To optimize efforts in the future, provide a debriefing after each course scenario and after each real resuscitation attempt.

What to say when local protocols for the use of a bag-mask device differ from what the course teaches:

In the course, you learned about providing ventilation with a bag-mask device. Your local protocol may call for chest compressions only, 200 chest compressions before breaths, use of a bag-mask device with a face mask for a short time until a supraglottic airway can be placed (as soon as possible), or a variation of these.

- Follow the local protocol.
- Provide only enough volume with each ventilation to make the chest rise (do not deliver large breaths that can potentially inhibit venous blood flow back into the chest).
- When delivering ventilation during CPR with an advanced airway, provide no more than 12 breaths per minute (excessive ventilation can increase intrathoracic pressure, impede venous return, and potentially reduce cerebral blood flow).
- Do not interrupt chest compressions for extended lengths of time to place an advanced or supraglottic airway.

Lesson 7
Child BLS

10 minutes

Part 1: Pediatric Chains of Survival

Part 2: Child BLS

Part 3: 2-Rescuer Child CPR (Practice While Watching)

Learning Objective

Tell students that at the end of this lesson, they will be able to perform high-quality CPR for a child.

Instructor Tips

- Remind students to use their mobile phones to activate the emergency response system, if applicable.
- If you are using adult manikins for the child BLS practice, inform students that they may need to use 2 hands while practicing CPR because it's difficult to compress the adult manikin with 1 hand.
- Remind students that the technique used for child CPR will depend on the size of the child and the physical ability of the person performing compressions.
- Select a provider option to play for this lesson: in-facility or prehospital.
- To review this lesson, students can refer to Part 6: BLS for Infants and Children in the provider manual.

Play Video

The video will show and discuss the scenario, the pediatric Chains of Survival, and child BLS, including 2-rescuer child CPR and the differences between adult and child BLS:

- Witnessed vs unwitnessed if you are a single rescuer:
  - Witnessed: Immediately activate emergency response system and get an AED
  - Unwitnessed: If you are alone and must leave to activate the emergency response system, perform 5 cycles of CPR before leaving
- Compression depth: Compress approximately 2 inches (5 cm) or at least one third the depth of the chest
- Using 1 or 2 hands for child compressions: Use whichever allows you to provide deep, effective compressions
- Compression-to-ventilation ratio: 1-rescuer ratio is 30:2, and 2-rescuer ratio is 15:2

Video Pauses

- Ask students to position themselves at the side of their manikins.
- Tell them that they will practice each role of the 2-rescuer child BLS sequence. Assign students to play Rescuer 1 and Rescuer 2.
- After the first practice-while-watching segment, repeat the video for students to switch and practice the duties of the other role. Each student will complete 3 sets of 15:2.

Practice While Watching: 2-Rescuer Child CPR

Before playing the video, tell students to follow along with the video and complete the following steps:

Rescuer 1

- Ask Rescuer 1 to get into position at the victim's side to practice chest compressions. The student should
  - Compress at least one third the depth of the chest, approximately 2 inches (5 cm)
  - Compress at a rate of 100 to 120/min
  - Allow complete chest recoil after each compression without leaning on the chest between compressions
  - Minimize interruptions in compressions (try to limit any interruptions in chest compressions to less than 10 seconds)
  - Use a compression-to-ventilation ratio of 15:2
  - Count compressions out loud

Rescuer 2

- Ask Rescuer 2 to get into position at the victim's head and maintain an open airway. The student should
  - Perform a head tilt–chin lift or jaw thrust
  - Give breaths with a bag-mask device, watching for chest rise and avoiding excessive ventilation
- Tell Rescuer 2 to encourage Rescuer 1 to perform compressions that are deep enough and fast enough and to allow complete chest recoil after each compression.
- Emphasize the core concepts: push hard, push fast; allow complete chest recoil after each compression; when giving breaths, watch for chest rise; minimize interruptions in compressions (trying to limit any interruptions in chest compressions to less than 10 seconds).

Repeat Segment

Ask students to switch roles and repeat the practice-while-watching segment.

Skills Test (Optional)

You have the option to administer the Adult CPR and AED Skills Test now. If you choose to administer the skills test now, refer to Lesson 11: Skills Test in the BLS Lesson Plans.

Lesson 8
Infant BLS

20 minutes

Part 1: Infant BLS

Part 2: Infant Compressions (Practice While Watching)

Part 3: Bag-Mask Device for Infants (Practice While Watching)

Part 4: 2-Rescuer Infant CPR (Practice While Watching)

Part 5: AED for Infants and Children Less Than 8 Years of Age

Learning Objective

Tell students that at the end of this lesson, they will be able to perform high-quality CPR for an infant.

Instructor Tips

- Select a provider option to play for this lesson: in-facility or prehospital.
- To review this lesson, students can refer to Part 6: BLS for Infants and Children and Part 7: Automated External Defibrillator for Infants and Children Younger Than 8 Years of Age in the provider manual.

Play Video

The video will show and discuss the scenario, infant BLS, and infant compressions.

Video Pauses

- Ask students to position themselves at the side of their manikins.
- Tell them that they will practice infant chest compressions and complete 3 sets of 30 compressions.

Practice While Watching: Infant Compressions

Before playing the video, tell students to follow along with the video and complete the steps for infant compressions. Tell students the following:

- Place the infant on a firm, flat surface.
- Place 2 fingers in the center of the infant's chest, just below the nipple line, on the lower half of the breastbone. If students prefer, they can use the 2 thumb–encircling hands technique. Do not press the tip of the breastbone.
- Push hard and fast at a depth of at least one third the depth of the chest, approximately 1½ inches (4 cm). Deliver compressions at a rate of 100 to 120/min. If the student cannot achieve the recommended depth, you can tell the student that it may be reasonable to use the heel of 1 hand.
- Allow complete chest recoil after each compression without leaning on the chest between compressions.

- Minimize interruptions in compressions (trying to limit any interruptions in chest compressions to less than 10 seconds).

Play Video

The video will show and discuss bag-mask devices for infants.

Video Pauses

- Ask students to position themselves at the side of their manikins.
- Tell them that they will practice using the bag-mask device for infants. Each student will complete 5 sets of 2 breaths.

Practice While Watching: Bag-Mask Device for Infants

Before playing the video, tell students to follow along with the video and complete the steps for using a bag-mask device for infants. Tell students the following:

- Position yourself directly above the victim's head.
- Place the mask on the victim's face, using the bridge of the nose as a guide for correct position.
- Use the E-C clamp technique to hold the mask in place while you lift the jaw to hold the airway open.
  - Perform a head tilt–chin lift.
  - Place the mask on the face, with the narrow portion at the bridge of the nose.
  - Use the thumb and index finger of one hand to form a C on the side of the mask, pressing the edges of the mask to the face.
  - Use the remaining fingers to lift the angles of the jaw (3 fingers form an E), open the airway, and press the face to the mask.
- Squeeze the bag to give breaths (1 second each) while watching for chest rise. Deliver each breath over 1 second, whether or not you use supplemental oxygen.
  - Make sure students give 2 breaths and watch for chest rise.

Play Video

The video will show and discuss 2-rescuer infant CPR.

Video Pauses

- Ask students to position themselves at the side of their manikins.
- Tell students that they will practice each role of the 2-rescuer infant CPR sequence. Assign students to play Rescuer 1 and Rescuer 2.
- After the first practice-while-watching segment, the video will repeat for students to switch and practice the duties of the other role. Each student will complete 3 sets of 15:2.

Practice While Watching: 2-Rescuer Infant CPR

Before playing the video, tell students to follow along with the video and complete the following actions:

Rescuer 1

Ask Rescuer 1 to get into position by the victim's feet to practice the 2 thumb–encircling hands technique for providing chest compressions:

- Compress at least one third the depth of the infant's chest, approximately 1½ inches (4 cm).
- Compress at a rate of 100 to 120/min.
- Allow complete chest recoil after each compression without leaning on the chest between compressions.
- Minimize interruptions in compressions (trying to limit any interruptions in chest compressions to less than 10 seconds).
- Use a compression-to-ventilation ratio of 15:2.
- Count compressions out loud.

Rescuer 2

Have Rescuer 2 get into position at the victim's head and maintain an open airway. The student should

- Perform a head tilt–chin lift or jaw thrust
- Give breaths with a bag-mask device, watching for chest rise and avoiding excessive ventilation

Tell Rescuer 2 to encourage Rescuer 1 to perform compressions that are deep enough and fast enough and to allow complete chest recoil after each compression. Emphasize core concepts: push hard, push fast; allow complete chest recoil after each compression; when giving breaths, watch for chest rise; minimize interruptions in compressions (try to limit any interruptions in chest compressions to less than 10 seconds).

Repeat Segment

Ask students to switch roles and repeat the practice-while-watching segment.

Play Video

The video will show and discuss AED use for infants and children less than 8 years of age.

Students Practice: High-Performance Teams Activity

For additional student practice with high-performance teams, students can complete the high-performance teams activity by using an infant scenario. Refer to Lesson 6: High-Performance Teams in the BLS Lesson Plans for more on how to complete this activity with the following scenario:

"As part of a multirescuer emergency response team, you respond to a call from a parent who says her 9-month-old infant started having breathing difficulties after feeding."

Skills Test (Optional)

You have the option to administer the Infant CPR Skills Test now. If you choose to administer the skills test now, refer to Lesson 11: Skills Test in the BLS Lesson Plans. Remember that you may need the infant manikins for Lesson 9: Relief of Choking.

Lesson 9
Relief of Choking

7 minutes ●

Part 1: Adult and Child Choking

Part 2: Infant Choking (Practice While Watching)

Learning Objective

Tell students that at the end of this lesson, they will be able to describe the technique for relief of foreign-body airway obstruction for an adult, a child, and an infant.

Instructor Tips

- Select a provider option to play for this lesson: in-facility or prehospital.
- To review this lesson, students can refer to Part 11: Choking Relief for Adults, Children, and Infants in the provider manual.

Play Video

The video will show and discuss relief of choking in a responsive or an unresponsive adult or child.

Discussion

Ask students, "What questions do you have about choking relief for adults and children?" If needed, use the following to guide the discussion:

- What are signs of a severe airway obstruction?
- What actions should you take to help a person with a severe airway obstruction?
- How do you help a person with a severe airway obstruction who is pregnant, overweight, or can't stand?
- What should you do if the person becomes unresponsive?

Play Video

This video will show and discuss relief of choking in a responsive or an unresponsive infant.

Video Pauses

- Ask students to position themselves per the video instructions.
- Tell them that they will practice the relief of choking on a responsive infant and complete 1 set of 5 back slaps and 5 chest thrusts.

Practice While Watching: Relief of Choking in a Responsive Infant

Before playing the video, tell students to follow along with the video and complete the steps for relief of choking in a responsive infant. Tell students the following:

- Kneel or sit with the infant in your lap.
- If you can do it easily, remove clothing from the infant's chest.
- Hold the infant facedown, with the head slightly lower than the chest, resting on your forearm. Support the infant's head and jaw with your hand. Avoid compressing the soft tissues of the infant's throat. Rest your forearm on your lap or thigh to support the infant.
- Using the heel of your hand, deliver up to 5 back slaps forcefully between the infant's shoulder blades. Deliver each slap with enough force to dislodge the foreign body.
- After delivering up to 5 back slaps, place your free hand on the infant's back, supporting the back of the infant's head with the palm of your hand. The infant will be cradled adequately between your 2 forearms, with the palm of one hand supporting the face and jaw while the palm of the other hand supports the back of the infant's head.
- Turn the infant over while carefully supporting the head and neck. Hold the infant faceup, with your forearm resting on your thigh. Keep the infant's head lower than the trunk.
- Provide up to 5 quick downward chest thrusts in the middle of the chest, over the lower half of the breastbone (the same as for chest compressions during CPR). Deliver chest thrusts at a rate of about 1 per second with enough force to dislodge the foreign body.
- Repeat the sequence of up to 5 back slaps and up to 5 chest thrusts until the object is removed or the infant becomes unresponsive.
  - If the infant becomes unresponsive, activate the emergency response system. Start CPR with the additional step of checking the airway for a foreign object after each set of compressions.

Stop Video

Ask students to return to their seats for the conclusion of the course.

Lesson 10
Conclusion

Instructor Tips

- When summarizing what was covered in the course, allow students to lead the discussion. Ask 1 or 2 students what they observed or learned during the course.

- Explain to students the importance of skills practice on an ongoing basis. Evidence shows that when providers take standardized resuscitation courses, whether online or in person, their skills decay over time. Give students clear directions on specific actions to take for further study, including AHA resources for postclassroom training.

Discussion

Conclude the course by doing the following:

- Thank students for their participation.

- Summarize what they learned during the course. Refer to the BLS Course Outline in Part 3: Teaching the Course.

- Ask students if they have any questions before the exam.

- Make sure that students complete their evaluation forms.

- Collect all completed forms.

Optional: The Adult CPR and AED Skills Test also can be completed at the end of Lesson 7: Child BLS and the Infant CPR Skills Test can be completed at the end of Lesson 8: Infant BLS in the BLS Renewal Lesson Plans.

Part 1: Adult CPR and AED Skills Test

Part 2: Infant CPR Skills Test

Instructor Tips

- For skills testing, be prepared and organized by reviewing the skills testing checklists before class. Have all materials ready to properly test students on every step.

- Make sure students review the skills testing checklist before skills testing.

Discussion

Before the Adult CPR and AED Skills Test, read the following script aloud to each student or to the whole class at once:

"This test is like a real emergency: you should do whatever you think is necessary to save the victim's life. You will have to determine for yourself what you need to do. For example, if you check for a response on the manikin and there is no response, then you should do whatever you would do for a person who is not responding. I will read a short scenario to you, but I can't answer any questions. You can treat me like another healthcare provider who has arrived with you and tell me to do something to help you. If you make a mistake or forget to do something important, don't stop. Just do your best to correct the error. Continue doing what you would do in an actual emergency until I tell you to stop. Do you have any questions before we start?"

Skills Test

- Refer to the Adult CPR and AED Skills Testing Checklist in Part 4: Testing for directions on how to test students on adult BLS skills. Check off each skill as the student demonstrates competency per the critical skills descriptors.

- After starting, if the student asks any questions about BLS skills or sequences, do not answer. Rather, tell the student, "Do what you think is best right now." If the student asks questions about what to do with the manikin, say, "Check the manikin yourself and do what you think is needed to save a life." If the student seems unsure, reiterate that he or she will be assessing the manikin and doing whatever is necessary.

Discussion

Before the Infant CPR Skills Test, read the following script aloud to the student or to all students at once:

"This test is like a real emergency: you should do whatever you think is necessary to save the victim's life. You will have to determine for yourself what you need to do. For example, if you check the response on the manikin and there is no response, then you should do whatever you would do for a person who is not responding. I will read a short scenario to you, but I can't answer any questions. You can treat me like another healthcare provider who has arrived with you and tell me to do something to help you. If you make a mistake or forget to do something important, don't stop. Just do your best to correct the error. Continue doing what you would do in an actual emergency until I tell you to stop. Do you have any questions before we start?"

 ## Skills Test

- Refer to the Infant CPR Skills Testing Checklist in Part 4: Testing for directions on how to test students on infant BLS skills. Check off each skill as the student demonstrates competency per the critical skills descriptors.

- After starting, if the student asks any questions about BLS skills or sequences, do not answer. Rather, tell the student, "Do what you think is best right now." If the student asks questions about what to do with the manikin, tell the student, "Check the manikin yourself and do what you think is needed to save a life." If the student seems unsure, reiterate that he or she will be assessing the manikin and doing whatever is necessary.

Remediation

For students who need remediation, follow these steps, and refer to Lesson 13: Remediation in the BLS Lesson Plans:

- Determine where the student is having trouble during their Adult CPR and AED Skills Test and/or Infant CPR Skills Test.

- If needed, replay sections of video or practice skills to reinforce learning.

- Retest skills as necessary.

- Some students may need additional practice or to repeat the course to demonstrate skills competency and receive a course completion card.

Lesson 12
Exam

25 minutes

Instructor Tips

- Exams are administered online, though there may be an occasional need to administer a paper exam. Refer to the Instructor Network for more information about delivering exams.
- You should administer the exam after skills testing at the end of the course.
- During testing and remediation, assign each additional instructor a different role, especially with large classes. This will help remediation be efficient and effective. This also will help the class end on time.
- For the exam, provide students with an environment that's conducive to testing: quiet, with minimal distractions and plenty of time to finish.

Discussion

Give students the following instructions:

- For students taking a paper exam: Do not write on the exam. Write only on your answer sheet.
- Do not cooperate with or talk to each other during the exam.
- Exams are open resource, so you can use the provider manual and any other accessible resources while taking the exam.

Refer to Part 1: General Concepts for details about open-resource exams.

Exam

- For students taking a paper exam: Distribute answer sheets and exams.
- As students finish, collect their exams and answer sheets and begin to grade them.
- Regardless of their scores, all students should receive their exam results so that they can review and ask questions.

Remediation

For students who need remediation, refer to Lesson 13: Remediation in the BLS Lesson Plans.

Lesson 13
Remediation

15 minutes ●

Part 1: Skills Testing Remediation
Part 2: Exam Remediation

Instructor Tips

- Use the formal remediation lesson if a student did not pass the skills testing during the course.
- For further detail on remediation and retesting students, refer to Part 1: General Concepts.
- As an instructor, you will need to determine which section of the course the student is having trouble with.

Play Video: Skills Testing Remediation

- Replay instruction and/or practice-while-watching segments of the video as needed to reinforce learning and for the student to have additional practice.
- Repeat practice until the student feels comfortable and is ready to move forward with the skills test.
  - Some students may need additional practice or to repeat the course to demonstrate skills competency and receive a course completion card.
- Formal remediation should occur if all boxes on the skills testing checklist are not checked as complete.

Skills Test

- Retest BLS skills as necessary by using the skills testing checklists. Refer to Lesson 11 in the BLS Lesson Plans for additional instructions on administering the skills tests.

Exam

Students who are taking the paper exam and score less than 84% need immediate remediation and must retake the exam.

- Provide remediation by giving a second test or by having students verbally answer each item they answered incorrectly, showing an understanding of the incorrect items.
- Give students their failed exams to study in preparation for retaking the exam.
- After successful remediation, students should show improvement in providing and understanding correct responses.
- Collect all exams and answer sheets from all students at the end of the course or after remediation.

Postcourse
Immediately After the Course

At the end of each class

- Collect, organize, and check all course paperwork for completeness
- Rearrange the room
- Clean and store equipment
- Fill out Training Center course report forms
- Read and consider comments from course evaluations
- Conduct a debriefing with assisting staff
- Issue eCards according to Training Center policy; if you are unsure of the policy, check with the Training Center Coordinator

Reminder: To ensure that students receive their course completion cards within 20 business days after completing a class, submit the paperwork to your Training Center as soon as possible after the class.

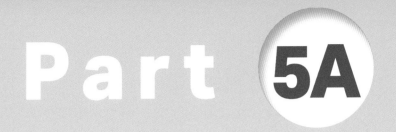

BLS Renewal Lesson Plans

Precourse Preparation

Instructor Tips

Prepare well for your role as a BLS Instructor. Review all course materials and anticipate questions or challenges that may arise during the course. The time you invest in this preparation is important to the overall success of every student.

Refer to Part 3: Teaching the Course in the instructor manual for further instructions on using lesson plans.

30 to 60 Days Before the Course

- Determine course specifics, such as
  - Your students' professions (in-facility or prehospital providers) and how they'll use the skills you teach in this course at work
  - Number of participating students
  - Any special equipment needed for the course
- Reserve all the equipment you need for the course. Refer to Part 2: Preparing for the Course in the instructor manual for a complete equipment list.
- Schedule a room that meets the requirements for the BLS Renewal Course. Refer to Part 2: Preparing for the Course in the instructor manual for details.
- Schedule additional instructors, if needed, depending on your class size.

At Least 3 Weeks Before the Course

- Send participating students the precourse letter, the course agenda, and student materials.
- Confirm any additional scheduled instructors.
- Research your local protocols, and encourage students to know them before coming to class. This will help you answer students' questions during the course. Refer to optional Lesson 4A: Local Protocols Discussion in the BLS Renewal Lesson Plans for more details and examples.
- Confirm that all students have the required prerequisite: a current BLS Provider course completion card.

Day Before the Course

- Confirm room reservations and ensure that all required equipment is available.
- Set up the room and make sure that all technology and equipment work. You can do this the day of the course if the room is not accessible the day before.
- Locate the nearest AED in the building and confirm the emergency response number.
- Coordinate all roles and responsibilities with any additional instructors to ensure efficiency and timing, per the course agenda.
- Ensure that all course paperwork is in order.
- If you will be using the Full Code Pro app for the high-performance teams activity, download the app to an iOS smartphone or tablet. Review the app before class to become familiar with the functionality.

Day of the Course

Arrive at the course location in plenty of time to complete the following:

- Make sure all equipment works and has been cleaned according to manufacturer instructions.
- Have the video ready to play before students arrive.
- Distribute supplies or set them out for students to collect, and offer clear instructions on what they need.
- Greet students as they arrive to put them at ease, and direct them where to go.
- Make sure students complete the course roster as they arrive.

Lesson 1
Course Introduction

5 minutes

Instructor Tips

- Be familiar with the learning objectives and BLS Course content. It's critical that you know what you want to communicate, why it's important, and what you want to happen as a result.

- Prebrief the students. Explain that this is a safe space for learning and that mistakes are expected as part of the learning process. Students can practice skill repetition with your feedback to improve their performance. Remind students that they must demonstrate mastery of key resuscitation skills to successfully complete the course.

- Tailor the learning experience to students' real-world scope of practice, if possible. Consider the types of students, their settings, and the resources that are available to them. Structure team training so that scenarios, team composition, and roles are relevant.

- Think about how you'll manage breaks during the course. Consider using the time to establish rapport, get feedback, and answer questions students might feel too embarrassed to ask in front of everyone.

 ## Discussion

- Introduce yourself and any additional instructors.

- Invite students to introduce themselves.

- Explain that the course is interactive. Discuss your role, video-based learning, the provider manual, the scenarios, practice while watching, and skills tests and the exam.
  - Refer to Part 3: Teaching the Course for detailed information about practice while watching.

- Ask students to speak to an instructor if they anticipate difficulties due to medical concerns, such as knee or back problems. Refer to Part 1: General Concepts for more about students with special needs.

- Explain the layout of the building, including bathrooms and emergency exits.

- Tell students the location of the nearest AED and the emergency response number.

- Describe the course agenda, including when you'll have breaks and when the class will end.

- Remind students that at the end of the BLS Course, they will be able to
  - Describe the importance of high-quality CPR and its impact on survival
  - Describe all of the steps of the Chain of Survival
  - Apply the BLS concepts of the Chain of Survival
  - Recognize the signs of someone needing CPR
  - Perform high-quality CPR for an adult, a child, and an infant
  - Describe the importance of using an AED as soon as possible
  - Demonstrate the appropriate use of an AED
  - Provide effective ventilation by using a barrier device

- – Describe the importance of teams in multirescuer resuscitation attempts
- – Perform as an effective team member during multirescuer CPR
- – Describe the techniques for relief of foreign-body airway obstruction for an adult, a child, and an infant
- For further detail on the video and scenarios to be shown during the course, refer to the BLS Course Outline in Part 3: Teaching the Course.
- Remind students that to complete the course, they must
  - – Pass the Adult CPR and AED Skills Test
  - – Pass the Infant CPR Skills Test
  - – Score at least 84% on the exam

Lesson 2
Adult BLS

22 minutes

Part 1: Adult Chains of Survival

Part 2: 1-Rescuer Adult BLS (Practice While Watching)

Part 3: AED Practice (Students Practice)

Part 4: Bag-Mask Device (Practice While Watching)

Learning Objectives

Tell students that at the end of this lesson, they will be able to

- Describe the importance of high-quality CPR and its impact on survival
- Describe all of the steps of the Chain of Survival
- Apply the BLS concepts of the Chain of Survival
- Recognize the signs of someone needing CPR
- Perform high-quality CPR for an adult
- Describe the importance of using an AED as soon as possible
- Demonstrate the appropriate use of an AED

Instructor Tips

- Remind students that they will be practicing while watching a video segment so that they are prepared to get into place quickly to practice.

- When students are practicing, focus your feedback on what you do want rather than what you don't want. Always state feedback in a positive tone.

- Tell students to have their provider manuals accessible during the course.

- When concluding a practice-while-watching session, ask students if they are ready to move to the next skill or if they would like to repeat practice while watching.

- Learn how to assemble and operate all of the equipment that students will use in class. Be prepared to help them with it as needed and troubleshoot any problems.

- Select a provider option to play for this lesson: in-facility or prehospital.

- To review this lesson, students can refer to Part 3: BLS for Adults in the provider manual.

Play Video

The video will show and discuss the adult Chains of Survival and 1-rescuer adult BLS.

Video Pauses

- Have students position themselves at the side of their manikins per the video instructions.

- Tell them that they will practice the entire 1-rescuer adult BLS sequence, including scene safety and assessment and 3 sets of 30 compressions, with 2 breaths at the end of each set of compressions.

- Tell students to compress at a rate of 100 to 120/min, making sure compressions are at least 2 inches (5 cm) deep and allowing complete chest recoil.

 # Practice While Watching: 1-Rescuer Adult BLS

Students will follow along with the video to complete the steps for scene safety and assessment, adult compressions, and pocket mask use. For all video segments, repeat the practice-while-watching segment as many times as needed for all students to complete the practice session.

Scene Safety and Assessment

Before playing the video, tell students to follow along with the video and complete the steps for scene safety and assessment. Tell students the following:

- Verify that the scene is safe for you and the victim.
- Check for responsiveness. Tap the victim's shoulder and shout, "Are you OK?"
- If the victim is not responsive, shout for nearby help.
- Assess the victim for the presence of a pulse and normal breathing.
- Activate the emergency response system in your setting.
- Get the AED. If someone else is available, have that person get it.

Adult Compressions

Before playing the video, tell students to follow along with the video and complete the steps for adult compressions. Tell students the following:

- Position yourself at the victim's side.
- Put the heel of one hand on the center of the victim's chest, on the lower half of the breastbone (sternum).
- Put the heel of your other hand on top of the first hand.
- Straighten your arms and position your shoulders directly over your hands.
- Give chest compressions:
  - Press down at least 2 inches (5 cm) with each compression. Make sure you push straight down on the victim's breastbone.
  - Deliver compressions at a rate of 100 to 120/min.
  - Allow complete chest recoil after each compression without leaning on the chest between compressions.
- Minimize interruptions in chest compressions (trying to limit any interruptions in chest compressions to less than 10 seconds).

Emphasize core concepts: Use correct hand placement, push hard and fast, allow complete chest recoil after each compression, and minimize pauses in compressions.

Pocket Mask

Before playing the video, tell students to follow along with the video and complete the steps for using a pocket mask. Tell students the following:

- Position yourself at the victim's side.
- Place the pocket mask on the victim's face, using the bridge of the nose as a guide for correct position.

- Seal the pocket mask against the face:
  - Using your hand that is closer to the top of the victim's head, place the index finger and thumb along the edge of the mask that is on the nose.
  - Place the thumb of your other hand along the edge of the mask that is on the chin.
- Place the remaining fingers of your second hand along the bony margin of the jaw and lift the jaw. Perform a head tilt–chin lift to open the airway.
- While you lift the jaw, press firmly and completely around the outside edge of the mask to seal the pocket mask against the face.
- Deliver each breath over 1 second, enough to make the victim's chest rise.
- Tell students to hold the mask firmly against the face. Emphasize visible chest rise.
- To review this portion of the lesson, students can refer to Part 4: Automated External Defibrillator for Adults and Children 8 Years of Age and Older and Part 3: BLS for Adults in the provider manual.

Play Video

The video will show and discuss AED use, including AED special considerations, such as if the person

- Has a hairy chest
- Is immersed in water or has water covering the chest
- Has an implanted defibrillator or pacemaker
- Has a transdermal medication patch or other object on the surface of the skin where the AED pads need to be placed
- Is an infant or child less than 8 years of age
- Is a pregnant woman

Video Pauses: AED Review

During the pause, show students the AED trainer and

- Explain how to use the AED trainer; remind students that it will not deliver a real shock
- Emphasize following the AED prompts
- Direct students to have their AED trainers out and ready to use
- Tell students that they are now going to practice using the AED

Students Practice: AED

Provide the following instructions on how to use an AED. First show the steps while using your AED trainer, and then ask students to practice.

Instructions for Students

1. Open the carrying case. Power on the AED if needed.
   - Some devices will power on automatically when you open the lid or case.
   - Follow the AED prompts for the next steps.
2. Attach AED pads to the victim's bare chest.
   - Choose adult pads (not child pads or a child system) for victims 8 years of age and older.
   - Peel the backing from the AED pads.
   - Attach the adhesive AED pads to the victim's bare chest. Place one pad on the manikin's upper-right chest (directly below the collarbone). Place the other pad to the side of the left nipple, with the top edge of the pad a few inches below the armpit.
   - Attach the AED connecting cables to the AED box (some are preconnected).
3. Clear the manikin and analyze the rhythm.
   - If the AED prompts you, clear the victim during analysis. Be sure no one is touching the victim, not even the rescuer in charge of giving breaths.
   - Some AEDs will tell you to push a button to allow the AED to begin analyzing the heart rhythm; others will do that automatically. The AED may take a few seconds to analyze.
   - The AED then tells you if a shock is needed.
4. If the AED advises a shock, it will tell you to clear the victim.
   - Clear the victim before delivering the shock; be sure no one is touching the victim.
   - Loudly state a "clear the victim" message, such as "Everybody clear" or simply "Clear."
   - Look to be sure no one is in contact with the victim.
   - Press the shock button.
5. The shock will produce a sudden contraction of the victim's muscles.
6. If the AED prompts that no shock is advised, or after any shock is delivered, immediately resume CPR, starting with chest compressions.

 ## Play Video

The video will show and discuss bag-mask devices.

 ## Video Pauses

- Ask students to position themselves at the side of their manikins.
- Tell them that they will practice using the bag-mask device and complete 5 sets of 2 breaths.

 ## Practice While Watching: Bag-Mask Device

Before playing the video, tell students to follow along with the video and complete the steps for using a bag-mask device. Tell students the following:

- Position yourself directly above the victim's head.
- Place the mask on the victim's face, using the bridge of the nose as a guide for correct position.

- Use the E-C clamp technique to hold the mask in place while you lift the jaw to hold the airway open.
  - Perform a head tilt–chin lift.
  - Place the mask on the face, with the narrow portion at the bridge of the nose.
  - Use the thumb and index finger of one hand to form a C on the side of the mask, pressing the edges of the mask to the face.
  - Use the remaining fingers to lift the angles of the jaw (3 fingers form an E), open the airway, and press the face to the mask.
- Squeeze the bag to give breaths (1 second each) while watching for chest rise. Deliver each breath over 1 second, whether or not you use supplemental oxygen.
  - Instructors: Make sure students give 2 breaths and watch for chest rise.

Lesson 3
Special Considerations

10 minutes

Part 1: Mouth-to-Mouth Breaths

Part 2: Rescue Breathing (Practice While Watching)

Part 3: Breaths With an Advanced Airway

Part 4: Opioid-Associated Life-Threatening Emergency

Part 5: Maternal Cardiac Arrest

Instructor Tips

- Select a provider option to play for this lesson: in-facility or prehospital.

- To review this lesson, students can refer to Part 8: Alternate Ventilation Techniques and Part 9: Opioid-Associated Life-Threatening Emergencies in the provider manual.

Play Video

The video will show and discuss mouth-to-mouth breaths and rescue breathing.

Video Pauses

- Ask students to position themselves at the side of their manikins.

- Tell them that they will practice rescue breathing on the manikin.

- You may ask students to practice rescue breathing on infant manikins instead of adult manikins. If selecting this option, go to Students Practice: Rescue Breathing (Infants and Children) instead of Practice While Watching: Rescue Breathing (Adults).

Practice While Watching: Rescue Breathing (Adults)

Before playing the video, tell students to follow along with the video and complete the steps for adult rescue breathing. Tell students the following:

- Give 1 breath every 6 seconds.

- Give each breath over 1 second, ensuring that each breath results in visible chest rise.

- Check the pulse about every 2 minutes.

Students Practice: Rescue Breathing (Infants and Children)

Discuss and then ask students to practice the steps for providing rescue breathing for infants and children. Tell students the following:

- Give 1 breath every 2 to 3 seconds (about 20 to 30 breaths per minute).

- Give each breath over 1 second.

- Each breath should result in visible chest rise.

- Check the pulse about every 2 minutes

Play Video

The video will show and discuss breaths with an advanced airway, opioid-associated life-threatening emergencies, and maternal cardiac arrest.

- Advanced airway
    - No pauses in compressions
    - Adults: 1 breath every 6 seconds
    - Children and infants: 1 breath every 2 to 3 seconds
- Opioid-associated life-threatening emergencies
    - In all instances of opioid-associated life-threating emergencies, activate emergency medical services
    - If the victim is breathing and has a pulse, monitor breathing and consider naloxone
    - If the victim is not breathing and has a pulse, provide rescue breathing and give naloxone
    - If the victim is not breathing and has no pulse, start CPR
- Maternal cardiac arrest
    - Compressions, ventilation, and AED use remain unchanged for a pregnant woman
    - Manual displacement of the rounded abdomen to mother's left side (lateral uterine displacement) should be done if enough rescuers are present to continue with CPR

Lesson 4
High-Performance Teams

26 minutes

Part 1: Team Dynamics

Part 2: High-Performance Teams

Part 3: High-Performance Teams Activity (Optional)

Learning Objective

Tell students that at the end of this lesson, they will be able to describe the importance of teams in multirescuer resuscitation.

Instructor Tips

- To engage students during discussion, ask open-ended questions that elicit students' own unique perspectives. This will help increase participation.

- When answering a question, make eye contact to acknowledge the student. Then, address the entire room. From time to time, direct your attention back to the student who asked the question.

- The Team Dynamics portion of this lesson focuses on the elements of effective team dynamics, including the roles everyone must play. The High-Performance Teams portion of the lesson focuses on the skills needed to achieve specific performance metrics, including a high CCF.

- CCF is the proportion of time that rescuers perform chest compressions during CPR. Shorter duration of interruptions in chest compressions is associated with better outcome. A CCF of at least 60% increases the likelihood of return of spontaneous circulation, shock success, and survival to hospital discharge. With good teamwork, rescuers can often achieve 80% CCF. In a 10-minute scenario, total chest compression time must be about 8 minutes to achieve an 80% CCF.

- Explain that BLS providers are responsible for performing only the roles on a resuscitation team that are within their training and scope of practice. It is important, however, to understand all team roles to be an effective team member.

- Select a provider option to play for this lesson: in-facility or prehospital.

- To review this lesson, students can refer to Part 5: Team Dynamics in the provider manual.

Play Video: Team Dynamics

The video will show and discuss good team dynamics; team roles, including Team Leader, Compressor, Airway, IV/IO/Medications, Monitor/Defibrillator/CPR Coach, and Timer/ Recorder; and the following information about successful resuscitation teams:

- The roles of each member
  - Clear roles and responsibilities
  - Knowing your limitations
  - Constructive intervention (be tactful)

- What to communicate
  - Knowledge sharing and frequently asking for observations
  - Summarizing and reevaluating, which can help respond to the patient's changing condition
- How to communicate
  - Closed-loop communication
  - Confirm order
  - Call people by their names
  - Confirm intervention complete
  - Clear messages
  - Speak in a calm, confident manner
  - Mutual respect
  - Behave in a professional manner
  - Use a friendly, controlled voice
  - Avoid shouting or aggression
- Debriefing
  - Debrief together as a team
  - Debrief after a resuscitation attempt
  - Debriefing may improve team performance and patient outcomes after cardiac arrest
- CPR Coach
  - The CPR Coach supports performance of high-quality BLS skills, allowing the Team Leader to focus on other aspects of clinical care. Studies have shown that resuscitation teams with a CPR Coach perform higher-quality CPR with higher CCF and shorter pause durations compared with teams that don't use a CPR Coach. This role was briefly covered in the Team Dynamics portion of this lesson.
  - The CPR Coach focuses only on compressions and ventilation to ensure high-quality CPR. They help minimize the length of pauses during provider switches and defibrillation.
  - The CPR Coach should be positioned next to the Defibrillator and in the direct line of sight of the Compressor.
  - Because the CPR Coach must continually talk to give ongoing coaching, they must adjust their tone and volume so that they do not disrupt other aspects of patient care.
  - The CPR Coach should respect the Team Leader's role and not be perceived as trying to take over leadership. They should keep the Team Leader informed, share their understanding with the Team Leader, and ask for verification of key tasks and decisions.
  - Any healthcare professional can be a CPR Coach if they have a current BLS Provider card, understand the responsibilities of a CPR Coach, and demonstrate the ability to coach Compressors and Airway providers effectively to improve performance.

Video Resumes: High-Performance Teams

The video will show and discuss the following information about the skills needed to achieve specific high-performance team metrics like CCF by eliminating the pauses commonly seen in a resuscitation attempt. Some key concepts covered include

- Hovering over the chest when compressions are paused
- Checking the pulse and precharging the defibrillator about 15 seconds before pausing compressions every 2 minutes
- Switching Compressors every 2 minutes or whenever a Compressor is fatigued, with the second Compressor coming in behind the first
- Using real-time feedback devices during CPR, or a metronome if a feedback device is not available

Play Video: High-Performance Teams Activity (Optional)

The video will show and discuss the high-performance teams activity.

Instructor Tips

- During this activity, watch the performance of multiple rescuers simultaneously. Take note of team performance that can be improved to inform topics of discussion during the debriefing. You will present one 10-minute scenario and follow with a 5-minute debriefing.
- While students practice, you will calculate the CCF.

How Do I Measure CCF?

Option 1: Use 2 stopwatches.

1. Start one stopwatch as soon as you give the scenario to the team. Let it run continuously to the 10-minute mark (total resuscitation time) as a reminder to stop the case.

2. Use a second stopwatch to measure total compression time during the scenario. Start the stopwatch each time a Compressor starts chest compressions. Pause the stopwatch when the Compressor stops or when chest compressions are interrupted. Do this for each set of compressions during the entire scenario. Don't reset the stopwatch during the scenario; allow the stopwatch to continue counting up. This will give you the cumulative time that chest compressions were being performed during the scenario.

3. Convert the time on the second stopwatch to seconds (eg, 8 minutes = 480 seconds).

4. Divide the total compression time in seconds by the total resuscitation time in seconds (ie, 10 minutes = 600 seconds).

5. This will give you the CCF. For example, if time on the second stopwatch is 520 seconds, divide by 600 (total resuscitation time): 520/600=0.8667. Then, round to 2 places and convert to a percentage: 87%.

Option 2: Use the AHA's Full Code Pro app. This app is a free, easy-to-use, mobile application that allows rescuers to document critical interventions during CPR. You can use Full Code Pro during real resuscitation events or in practice scenarios. Go to **https://itunes.apple.com/us/app/full-code-pro/id589451064?mt=8** to download the app for iOS devices. A Full Code Pro Tutorial video is available on the AHA Instructor Network.

Option 3: Use a manikin that captures resuscitation data.

Video Pauses

- Divide students into groups for the scenario. Assign team roles. Explain that after you read the scenario, students will begin the high-performance teams activity, which will run for 10 minutes. You will evaluate the resuscitation, looking for high-quality CPR and ensuring that students enforce the principles of highly effective teams. Briefly remind students that you will be tracking CCF because limiting interruptions in chest compressions improves outcome.

- Begin CCF tracking as soon as the Compressor begins chest compressions during CPR.

Students Practice

Read this scenario to each team:

- "As part of a multirescuer emergency response team, you respond to a call about a 65-year-old woman who suddenly collapsed. Your team arrives within seconds after the incident, and you notice that a bystander is performing compression-only CPR."

- Coach students in teamwork throughout the activity. Monitor CPR performance to inform high-quality CPR coaching, including minimizing pauses in compressions during the use of the AED. Provide focused practice as needed.

- Pay particular attention to the Compressor's performance toward the end of each 2-minute rotation. Monitor for high-quality compressions of adequate rate and depth. Remind the Compressor to allow complete chest recoil after each compression without leaning on the chest between compressions.

Discussion: High-Performance Teams Activity Debriefing

- At the end of the scenario, debrief by asking team members what they thought went well and what could have been better.
  - Disclose the CCF and discuss any strategies for improvement.
  - Talk about whether the team maintained high-quality CPR.
  - Allow the team to lead the conversation; ask open-ended questions to facilitate discussion.

- Coach on improving communication with closed-loop communication principles:
  - The Team Leader gives a message, an order, or an assignment to a team member.
  - The team member gives a clear response and makes eye contact to confirm that they heard and understood the message.
  - The Team Leader listens for confirmation of task performance from the team member before assigning another task.

Lesson 4A
Local Protocols Discussion (Optional)

20 minutes

Instructor Tips

- Across the country, EMS systems develop treatment protocols based on local need, preference of administration, and medical direction. In some cases, these protocols differ from established national standards, so this course may occasionally direct providers to act in ways that are not consistent with their local protocols. The AHA does not want to conflict with established local protocols.

- When you lead this discussion, make sure you know what the local protocols are. If you are a member of the local EMS system, you should already be aware of local protocols, but if you are not, study them before the course so that you can have a meaningful discussion.

Although the AHA does not endorse a particular protocol or strategy, it does issue evidence-based guidelines, which are relevant and broadly applicable. These guidelines are developed by experts in the field, who use a rigorous, scientific process. This discussion is a chance for students to articulate and practice AHA skills within the context of their local protocols.

Discussion

Lead students through a discussion about high-performance teams and local protocols. Use these questions to help guide this discussion:

- Does your system currently use a high-performance team approach to resuscitation?
- How can you incorporate high-performance teamwork into your department's protocols?
- What are some potential challenges to incorporating high-performance teamwork into your protocols?
- What are some potential challenges to high-performance teamwork in terms of location, patients, or equipment?
- How does the local protocol compare and contrast with the AHA BLS Healthcare Provider Adult Cardiac Arrest Algorithm?

The following examples show some common differences between local protocols and what is taught in the course. Use these sections only if students ask questions about these examples.

What to say when local protocols for chest compressions differ from what the course teaches:

In the course, you learned to do 30 high-quality chest compressions and then 2 breaths. This could differ from your local protocol, which may have you do 90 seconds of continuous chest compressions or 200 chest compressions before beginning breaths, or a variation of these.

- Follow the local protocol.
- The important factors in this lesson are to perform the compressions at a rate of 100 to 120/min, at least 2 inches in depth, while allowing the chest to recoil completely after each compression.
- The next Compressor should be immediately ready to switch roles to minimize interruption in compressions.

Studies show that patients who receive chest compressions at a rate of 100 to 120/min and a CCF of greater than 80% have a much better chance of survival.

What to say when local protocols for AED use differ from what the course teaches:

In the course, you learned to use the AED immediately after it arrives. This could differ from your local protocol, which may have you use the AED only after you do 200 chest compressions (or 2 minutes of CPR) or a variation of this.

- Follow the local protocol.
- Continue high-quality chest compressions up to the point of allowing the AED to analyze.
- Immediately begin chest compressions after a shock is delivered or the AED states, "no shock advised."
- Keep in mind that as time to defibrillation increases, the chance of survival decreases.

The greatest chance of survival from cardiac arrest is found when a patient receives high-quality CPR and early defibrillation.

What to say when local protocols for role assignment differ from what the course teaches:

In the course, you learned about the different roles that prehospital providers may have (Compressor, Timer/Recorder, etc). This could differ from your workplace protocol, which assigns you a role based on your role on the fire engine, ambulance, or other team.

- Follow the local protocol.
- Know your potential assignments ahead of time to reduce confusion during a real event.
- Make sure that all roles and responsibilities are clear so that interruptions in chest compressions are minimized and teamwork is smooth and efficient.
- It is critical that high-performance teams practice in the same way that they will perform in real situations.
- Appoint a Team Leader who oversees the event, assesses the efficacy of efforts, and makes changes when resuscitation performance is less than adequate.
- To optimize efforts in the future, provide a debriefing after each course scenario and after each real resuscitation attempt.

What to say when local protocols for the use of a bag-mask device differ from what the course teaches:

In the course, you learned about providing ventilation with a bag-mask device. Your local protocol may call for chest compressions only, 200 chest compressions before breaths, use of a bag-mask device with a face mask for a short time until a supraglottic airway can be placed (as soon as possible), or a variation of these.

- Follow the local protocol.
- Provide only enough volume with each ventilation to make the chest rise (do not deliver large breaths that can potentially inhibit venous blood flow back into the chest).
- When delivering ventilation during CPR with an advanced airway, provide no more than 12 breaths per minute (excessive ventilation can increase intrathoracic pressure, impede venous return, and potentially reduce cerebral blood flow).
- Do not interrupt chest compressions for extended lengths of time to place an advanced or supraglottic airway.

Lesson 5
Child BLS

9 minutes ●

Part 1: Pediatric Chains of Survival

Part 2: 2-Rescuer Child CPR (Practice While Watching)

Part 3: Adult CPR and AED Skills Test (Optional)

Learning Objective

Tell students that at the end of this lesson, they will be able to perform high-quality CPR for a child.

Instructor Tips

- Remind students to use their mobile phones to activate the emergency response system, if applicable.

- If you are using adult manikins for the child BLS practice, inform students that they may need to use 2 hands while practicing CPR because it's difficult to compress the adult manikin with 1 hand.

- Remind students that the technique used for child CPR will depend on the size of the child and the physical ability of the person performing compressions.

- Select a provider option to play for this lesson: in-facility or prehospital.

- To review this lesson, students can refer to Part 6: BLS for Infants and Children in the provider manual.

 ## Play Video

The video will show and discuss the pediatric Chains of Survival and 2-rescuer child CPR, including the differences between adult and child CPR:

- Witnessed vs unwitnessed if you are a single rescuer:

  – Witnessed: Immediately activate emergency response system and get an AED

  – Unwitnessed: If you are alone and must leave to activate the emergency response system, perform 5 cycles of CPR before leaving

- Compression depth: Compress approximately 2 inches or at least one third the depth of the chest

- Using 1 or 2 hands for child compressions: Use whichever allows you to provide deep, effective compressions

- Compression-to-ventilation ratio: 1-rescuer ratio is 30:2, and 2-rescuer ratio is 15:2

 ## Video Pauses

- Ask students to position themselves at the side of their manikins.

- Tell them that they will practice each role of the 2-rescuer child BLS sequence. Assign students to play Rescuer 1 and Rescuer 2.

- After the first practice-while-watching segment, repeat the video for students to switch and practice the duties of the other role. Each student will complete 3 sets of 15:2.

Practice While Watching: 2-Rescuer Child CPR

Before playing the video, tell students to follow along with the video and complete the following steps:

Rescuer 1

- Ask Rescuer 1 to get into position at the victim's side to practice chest compressions. The student should
  - Compress at least one third the depth of the chest, approximately 2 inches (5 cm)
  - Compress at a rate of 100 to 120/min
  - Allow complete chest recoil after each compression without leaning on the chest between compressions
  - Minimize interruptions in compressions (try to limit any interruptions in chest compressions to less than 10 seconds)
  - Use a compression-to-ventilation ratio of 15:2
  - Count compressions out loud

Rescuer 2

- Ask Rescuer 2 to get into position at the victim's head and maintain an open airway. The student should
  - Perform a head tilt–chin lift or jaw thrust
  - Give breaths with a bag-mask device, watching for chest rise and avoiding excessive ventilation
- Tell Rescuer 2 to encourage Rescuer 1 to perform compressions that are deep enough and fast enough and to allow complete chest recoil after each compression.
- Emphasize the core concepts: push hard, push fast; allow complete chest recoil after each compression; when giving breaths, watch for chest rise; minimize interruptions in compressions (trying to limit any interruptions in chest compressions to less than 10 seconds).

Repeat Segment

Ask students to switch roles and repeat the practice-while-watching segment.

Skills Test (Optional)

You have the option to administer the Adult CPR and AED Skills Test now. If you choose to administer the skills test now, refer to Lesson 9: Skills Test in the BLS Renewal Lesson Plans.

Lesson 6
Infant BLS

Part 1: Infant Compressions (Practice While Watching)

Part 2: 2-Rescuer Infant CPR (Practice While Watching)

Part 3: AED for Infants and Children Less Than 8 Years of Age

Part 4: Infant CPR Skills Test (Optional)

Learning Objective

Tell students that at the end of this lesson, they will be able to perform high-quality CPR for an infant.

Instructor Tips

- Select a provider option to play for this lesson: in-facility or prehospital.

- To review this lesson, students can refer to Part 6: BLS for Infants and Children and Part 7: Automated External Defibrillator for Infants and Children Younger Than 8 Years of Age in the provider manual.

Play Video

The video will show and discuss infant compressions.

Video Pauses

- Ask students to position themselves at the side of their manikins.

- Tell them that they will practice infant chest compressions and complete 3 sets of 30 compressions.

Practice While Watching: Infant Compressions

Before playing the video, tell students to follow along with the video and complete the steps for infant compressions. Tell students the following:

- Place the infant on a firm, flat surface.

- Place 2 fingers in the center of the infant's chest, just below the nipple line, on the lower half of the breastbone. Do not press the tip of the breastbone. If students prefer, they can use the 2 thumb–encircling hands technique.

- Push hard and fast at a depth of at least one third the depth of the chest, approximately 1½ inches (4 cm). Deliver compressions at a rate of 100 to 120/min. If the student cannot achieve the recommended depth, you can tell the student that it may be reasonable to use the heel of 1 hand.

- Allow complete chest recoil after each compression without leaning on the chest between compressions.

- Minimize interruptions in compressions (trying to limit any interruptions in chest compressions to less than 10 seconds).

Play Video

The video will show and discuss 2-rescuer infant CPR.

Video Pauses

- Ask students to position themselves at the side of their manikins.
- Tell students that they will practice each role of the 2-rescuer infant CPR sequence. Assign students to play Rescuer 1 and Rescuer 2.
- After the first practice-while-watching segment, the video will repeat for students to switch and practice the duties of the other role. Each student will complete 3 sets of 15:2.

Practice While Watching: 2-Rescuer Infant CPR

Before the video plays, tell students to follow along with the video and complete the following actions:

Rescuer 1

Ask Rescuer 1 to get into position by the victim's feet to practice the 2 thumb–encircling hands technique for providing chest compressions:

- Compress at least one third the depth of the infant's chest, approximately 1½ inches (4 cm).
- Compress at a rate of 100 to 120/min.
- Allow complete chest recoil after each compression without leaning on the chest between compressions.
- Minimize interruptions in compressions (trying to limit any interruptions in chest compressions to less than 10 seconds).
- Use a compression-to-ventilation ratio of 15:2.
- Count compressions out loud.

Rescuer 2

Have Rescuer 2 get into position at the victim's head and maintain an open airway. The student should

- Perform a head tilt–chin lift or jaw thrust
- Give breaths with a bag-mask device, watching for chest rise and avoiding excessive ventilation

Tell Rescuer 2 to encourage Rescuer 1 to perform compressions that are deep enough and fast enough and to allow complete chest recoil after each compression. Emphasize core concepts: push hard, push fast; allow complete chest recoil after each compression; when giving breaths, watch for chest rise; minimize interruptions in compressions (try to limit any interruptions in chest compressions to less than 10 seconds).

Repeat Segment

Ask students to switch roles and repeat the practice-while-watching segment.

Play Video

The video will show and discuss AED use for infants and children less than 8 years of age.

Students Practice: High-Performance Teams Activity

For additional student practice with high-performance teams, students can complete the high-performance teams activity by using an infant scenario. Refer to Lesson 4: High-Performance Teams in the BLS Renewal Lesson Plans for more on how to complete this activity with the following scenario:

"As part of a multirescuer emergency response team, you respond to a call from a parent who says her 9-month-old infant started having breathing difficulties after feeding."

Skills Test (Optional)

You have the option to administer the Infant CPR Skills Test now. If you choose to administer the skills test now, refer to Lesson 9: Skills Test in the BLS Renewal Lesson Plans. Remember that you may need the infant manikins for Lesson 7: Relief of Choking.

Lesson 7
Relief of Choking

7 minutes

Part 1: Adult and Child Choking

Part 2: Infant Choking (Practice While Watching)

Learning Objective

Tell students that at the end of this lesson, they will be able to describe the technique for relief of foreign-body airway obstruction for an adult, a child, and an infant.

Instructor Tips

- Select a provider option to play for this lesson: in-facility or prehospital.
- To review this lesson, students can refer to Part 11: Choking Relief for Adults, Children, and Infants in the provider manual.

 ## Play Video

The video will show and discuss relief of choking in a responsive or an unresponsive adult or child.

 ## Video Pauses

- Ask students to position themselves per the video instructions.
- Tell them that they will practice the relief of choking on a responsive infant and complete 1 set of 5 back slaps and 5 chest thrusts.

 ## Play Video

This video will show and discuss relief of choking in a responsive or an unresponsive infant.

 ## Practice While Watching: Relief of Choking in a Responsive Infant

Before playing the video, tell students to follow along with the video and complete the steps for relief of choking in a responsive infant. Tell students the following:

- Kneel or sit with the infant in your lap.
- If you can do it easily, remove clothing from the infant's chest.
- Hold the infant facedown, with the head slightly lower than the chest, resting on your forearm. Support the infant's head and jaw with your hand. Avoid compressing the soft tissues of the infant's throat. Rest your forearm on your lap or thigh to support the infant.
- Using the heel of your hand, deliver up to 5 back slaps forcefully between the infant's shoulder blades. Deliver each slap with enough force to dislodge the foreign body.
- After delivering up to 5 back slaps, place your free hand on the infant's back, supporting the back of the infant's head with the palm of your hand. The infant will be cradled adequately between your 2 forearms, with the palm of one hand supporting the face and jaw while the palm of the other hand supports the back of the infant's head.

- Turn the infant over while carefully supporting the head and neck. Hold the infant faceup, with your forearm resting on your thigh. Keep the infant's head lower than the trunk.
- Provide up to 5 quick downward chest thrusts in the middle of the chest, over the lower half of the breastbone (the same as for chest compressions during CPR). Deliver chest thrusts at a rate of about 1 per second with enough force to dislodge the foreign body.
- Repeat the sequence of up to 5 back slaps and up to 5 chest thrusts until the object is removed or the infant becomes unresponsive.
    - If the infant becomes unresponsive, activate the emergency response system. Start CPR with the additional step of checking the airway for a foreign object after each set of compressions.

 Stop Video

Ask students to return to their seats for the conclusion of the course.

Lesson 8
Conclusion

5 minutes

Instructor Tips

- When summarizing what was covered in the course, allow students to lead the discussion. Ask 1 or 2 students what they observed or learned during the course.

- Explain to students the importance of skills practice on an ongoing basis. Evidence shows that when providers take standardized resuscitation courses, whether online or in person, their skills decay over time. Give students clear directions on specific actions to take for further study, including AHA resources for postclassroom training.

Discussion

Conclude the course by doing the following:

- Thank students for their participation.

- Summarize what they learned during the course. Refer to the BLS Course Outline in Part 3: Teaching the Course.

- Ask students if they have any questions before the exam.

- Make sure that students complete their evaluation forms.

- Collect all completed forms.

Lesson 9
Skills Test

40 minutes ●

Optional: The Adult CPR and AED Skills Test also can be completed at the end of Lesson 5: Child BLS and the Infant CPR Skills Test can be completed at the end of Lesson 6: Infant BLS in the BLS Renewal Lesson Plans.

Part 1: Adult CPR and AED Skills Test

Part 2: Infant CPR Skills Test

Instructor Tips

- For skills testing, be prepared and organized by reviewing the skills testing checklists before class. Have all materials ready to properly test students on every step.

- Make sure students review the skills testing checklist before skills testing.

Discussion

Before the Adult CPR and AED Skills Test, read the following script aloud to each student or to the whole class at once:

"This test is like a real emergency: you should do whatever you think is necessary to save the victim's life. You will have to determine for yourself what you need to do. For example, if you check for a response on the manikin and there is no response, then you should do whatever you would do for a person who is not responding. I will read a short scenario to you, but I can't answer any questions. You can treat me like another healthcare provider who has arrived with you and tell me to do something to help you. If you make a mistake or forget to do something important, don't stop. Just do your best to correct the error. Continue doing what you would do in an actual emergency until I tell you to stop. Do you have any questions before we start?"

Skills Test

- Refer to the Adult CPR and AED Skills Testing Checklist in Part 4: Testing for directions on how to test students on adult BLS skills. Check off each skill as the student demonstrates competency per the critical skills descriptors.

- After starting, if the student asks any questions about BLS skills or sequences, do not answer. Rather, tell the student, "Do what you think is best right now." If the student asks questions about what to do with the manikin, say, "Check the manikin yourself and do what you think is needed to save a life." If the student seems unsure, reiterate that he or she will be assessing the manikin and doing whatever is necessary.

Discussion

Before the Infant CPR Skills Test, read the following script aloud to the student or to all students at once:

"This test is like a real emergency: you should do whatever you think is necessary to save the victim's life. You will have to determine for yourself what you need to do. For example, if you check the response on the manikin and there is no response, then you should do whatever you would do for a person who is not responding. I will read a short scenario to you, but I can't answer any questions. You can treat me like another healthcare provider who has arrived with you and tell me to do something to help you. If you make a mistake or forget to do something important, don't stop. Just do your best to correct the error. Continue doing what you would do in an actual emergency until I tell you to stop. Do you have any questions before we start?"

 ## Skills Test

- Refer to the Infant CPR Skills Testing Checklist in Part 4: Testing for directions on how to test students on infant BLS skills. Check off each skill as the student demonstrates competency per the critical skills descriptors.

- After starting, if the student asks any questions about BLS skills or sequences, do not answer. Rather, tell the student, "Do what you think is best right now." If the student asks questions about what to do with the manikin, tell the student, "Check the manikin yourself and do what you think is needed to save a life." If the student seems unsure, reiterate that he or she will be assessing the manikin and doing whatever is necessary.

Remediation

For students who need remediation, follow these steps, and refer to Lesson 11: Remediation in the BLS Renewal Lesson Plans:

- Determine where the student is having trouble during their Adult CPR and AED Skills Test and/or Infant CPR Skills Test.

- If needed, replay sections of video or practice skills to reinforce learning.

- Retest skills as necessary.

- Some students may need additional practice or to repeat the course to demonstrate skills competency and receive a course completion card.

Lesson 10
Exam

25 minutes

Instructor Tips

- Exams are administered online, though there may be an occasional need to administer a paper exam. Refer to the Instructor Network for more information about delivering exams.

- You should administer the exam after skills testing at the end of the course.

- During testing and remediation, assign each additional instructor a different role, especially with large classes. This will help remediation be efficient and effective. This also will help the class end on time.

- For the exam, provide students with an environment that's conducive to testing: quiet, with minimal distractions and plenty of time to finish.

Discussion

Give students the following instructions:

- For students taking a paper exam: Do not write on the exam. Write only on your answer sheet.

- Do not cooperate with or talk to each other during the exam.

- Exams are open resource, so you can use the provider manual and any other accessible resources while taking the exam.

Refer to Part 1: General Concepts for details about open-resource exams.

Exam

- For students taking a paper exam: Distribute answer sheets and exams.

- As students finish, collect their exams and answer sheet and begin to grade them.

- Regardless of their scores, all students should receive their exam results so that they can review and ask questions.

Remediation

For students who need remediation, refer to Lesson 11: Remediation in the BLS Renewal Lesson Plans.

Lesson 11
Remediation

15 minutes

- Part 1: Skills Testing Remediation
- Part 2: Exam Remediation

Instructor Tips

- Use the formal remediation lesson if a student did not pass the skills testing during the course.
- For further detail on remediation and retesting students, refer to Part 1: General Concepts.
- As an instructor, you will need to determine which section of the course the student is having trouble with.

Play Video: Skills Testing Remediation

- Replay instruction and/or practice-while-watching segments of the video as needed to reinforce learning and for the student to have additional practice.
- Repeat practice until the student feels comfortable and is ready to move forward with the skills test.
  - Some students may need additional practice or to repeat the course to demonstrate skills competency and receive a course completion card.
- Formal remediation should occur if all boxes on the skills testing checklist are not checked as complete.

Skills Test

- Retest BLS skills as necessary by using the skills testing checklists. Refer to Lesson 9 in the BLS Renewal Lesson Plans for additional instructions on administering the skills tests.

Exam

Students who are taking the paper exam and score less than 84% need immediate remediation and must retake the exam.

- Provide remediation by giving a second test or by having students verbally answer each item they answered incorrectly, showing an understanding of the incorrect items.
- Give students their failed exams to study in preparation for retaking the exam.
- After successful remediation, students should show improvement in providing and understanding correct responses.
- Collect all exams and answer sheets from all students at the end of the course or after remediation.

Postcourse
Immediately After the Course

At the end of each class:

- Collect, organize, and check all course paperwork for completeness.
- Rearrange the room.
- Clean and store equipment.
- Fill out Training Center course report forms.
- Read and consider comments from course evaluations.
- Conduct a debriefing with assisting staff.
- Issue eCards according to Training Center policy. If you are unsure of the policy, check with the Training Center Coordinator.
- Reminder: To ensure that students receive their course completion cards within 20 business days after completing a class, submit the paperwork to your Training Center as soon as possible after the class.

HeartCode® BLS Lesson Plans

Precourse Preparation

Instructor Tips

- Prepare for your role as a BLS Instructor well. Review all course materials and anticipate questions or challenges that may arise during the course. The time you invest in this part of your preparation is important to the overall success of every student.

- Refer to Part 2: Preparing for the Course for specific directions on preparing to teach blended-learning courses. Refer to Part 3: Teaching the Course for further instructions on using lesson plans.

30 to 60 Days Before Class

- Determine course specifics, such as
  - Your students' professions (in-facility or prehospital providers) and how they'll use the skills taught in this course
  - Number of students
  - Any special equipment needed for the course
- Reserve the equipment you need for the course. Refer to Part 2: Preparing for the Course for a complete equipment list.
- Schedule a room that meets BLS Course requirements. Refer to Part 2: Preparing for the Course for details.
- Schedule additional instructors, if needed, depending on your class size.

At Least 3 Weeks Before Class

- Send participating HeartCode BLS students their precourse letter, including the course key for the online portion, course agenda, and student materials.
- Confirm additional scheduled instructors, if needed.
- Research local protocols and encourage students to know them before coming to class. This will help you answer students' questions during the course. Refer to optional Lesson 5A: Local Protocols Discussion in the HeartCode BLS Lesson Plans for more details and examples.

Day Before Class

- Confirm room reservations and ensure that all required equipment is available.
- Set up the room and make sure that all technology and equipment work. You can do this the day of class if the room is not accessible the day before.
- Locate the nearest AED in the building and confirm the emergency response number.
- Coordinate all roles and responsibilities with any additional instructors to ensure efficiency and timing, per the course agenda.
- Ensure that all course paperwork is in order.
- If you will be using the Full Code Pro app for the high-performance teams activity, download the app to an iOS smartphone or tablet. Review the app before class to become familiar with the functionality.

Day of Class

Arrive at the course location in plenty of time to complete the following:

- Make sure that all equipment works and has been cleaned according to manufacturer instructions.
- Have the video ready to play before students arrive.
- Distribute supplies to the students or set up supplies for students to collect when they arrive, with clear instructions on what they need.
- Greet students as they arrive to put them at ease, and direct them where to go.
- Make sure students complete the course roster as they arrive.
- Collect each student's certificate of completion for the online portion of HeartCode BLS.

Lesson 1
Course Introduction

5 minutes

Instructor Tips

- Advise students that the course is fast-paced and allows students to watch and practice their skills.

- Be familiar with the learning objectives and BLS Course content. It's critical that you know what you want to communicate, why it's important, and what you want to happen as a result.

- Prebrief the students. Explain that this is a safe space for learning and that mistakes are expected as part of the learning process. Students can practice skill repetition with your feedback to improve their performance. Remind students that they must demonstrate mastery of key resuscitation skills to successfully complete the course.

- Tailor the learning experience to students' real-world scope of practice, if possible. Consider the types of students, their settings, and the resources that are available to them. Structure team training so that scenarios, team composition, and roles are relevant.

- Think about how you'll manage breaks during the course. Consider using the time to establish rapport, get feedback, and answer questions students might feel too embarrassed to ask in front of everyone.

 ## Discussion

- Introduce yourself and additional instructors, if present.

- Invite students to introduce themselves.

- Explain that the course is interactive. Refer to the following points (see detailed information for each throughout the instructor manual) for discussion with students:
  - Your role
  - Video-based learning
    - Review of each skill from the online portion of the course before skills practice
    - Practice while watching
      - Refer to Part 3: Teaching the Course for detailed information about practice while watching.
  - Skills test

- Ask students to speak to an instructor if they anticipate difficulties due to medical concerns, such as knee or back problems. Refer to Part 1: General Concepts for more about students with special needs.

- Explain the layout of the building, including bathrooms and emergency exits.

- Tell students the location of the nearest AED and the emergency response number.

- Describe the course agenda, including when you'll have breaks and when the class will end.

- Remind students what they will review and practice from the online portion during the classroom portion of the course. At the end of the HeartCode BLS Course, they will be able to
  - Describe the importance of high-quality CPR and its impact on survival
  - Describe all the steps of the Chain of Survival
  - Apply the BLS concepts of the Chain of Survival
  - Recognize the signs of someone needing CPR
  - Perform high-quality CPR for an adult, a child, and an infant
  - Describe the importance of using an AED as soon as possible
  - Demonstrate the appropriate use of an AED
  - Provide effective ventilation by using a barrier device
  - Describe the importance of teams in multirescuer resuscitation attempts
  - Perform as an effective team member during multirescuer CPR
  - Describe the techniques for relief of foreign-body airway obstruction for an adult, a child, and an infant
- For further detail on the video lessons to be shown during the course, refer to the HeartCode BLS Outline in Part 3: Teaching the Course.
- Remind students that to complete the course, they must
  - Pass the Adult CPR and AED Skills Test
  - Pass the Infant CPR Skills Test

Lesson 2
Adult BLS

27 minutes

At the beginning of this lesson, have students position themselves at the side of their manikins.

Part 1: Scene Safety, Assessment, and Adult Compressions

Part 2: Pocket Mask

Part 3: 1-Rescuer Adult BLS

Part 4: Bag-Mask Device

Part 5: 2-Rescuer Adult BLS

Learning Objectives

Tell students that at the end of this lesson, they will be able to

- Describe the importance of high-quality CPR and its impact on survival

- Apply the BLS concepts of the Chain of Survival

- Recognize the signs of someone needing CPR

- Perform high-quality CPR for an adult

- Provide effective ventilation by using a barrier device

- Perform as an effective team member during multirescuer CPR

Instructor Tips

- Video demonstration: Students will initially watch the video demonstrate a skill before the practice while watching.

- Practice while watching: After the demonstration, students will practice while watching along with the video segment. Notice the practice-while-watching icon that appears on the screen.

- Feedback: When providing feedback to students who are practicing, remember to focus on what you do want rather than what you don't want. Remember to always state feedback in a positive tone.

- When concluding a practice-while-watching session, ask students if they are ready to move to the next skill or if they would like to repeat practice while watching.

- Learn how to assemble and operate the equipment that students will use in class. Be prepared to help them with it as needed and troubleshoot any problems.

- Select a provider option to play for this lesson: in-facility or prehospital.

Play Video

The video will show and discuss

Demonstration: Scene Safety, Assessment, and Adult Compressions

- Ask students to position themselves at the side of their manikins to watch the demonstration.
- Tell them that they will practice being the first rescuer on the scene and checking for scene safety and assessing the victim after the demonstration.

Practice While Watching: Scene Safety, Assessment, and Adult Compressions

Scene Safety and Assessment

Before playing the video, tell students to follow along with the video and complete the actions for scene safety and assessment. Tell students the following:

- Verify that the scene is safe for you and the victim.
- Check for responsiveness. Tap the victim's shoulder and shout, "Are you OK?"
- If the victim is not responsive, shout for nearby help.
- Assess the victim for the presence of a pulse and normal breathing.
- Activate the emergency response system in your setting.
- Get the AED. If someone else is available, have that person get it.

You can also remind students that it's important to know where to find personal protective equipment in their work environment.

Adult Compressions

Before playing the video, tell students to follow along with the video and complete the steps for adult compressions. Tell students the following:

- Position yourself at the victim's side.
- Put the heel of one hand on the center of the victim's chest, on the lower half of the breastbone (sternum).
- Put the heel of your other hand on top of the first hand.
- Straighten your arms and position your shoulders directly over your hands.
- Give chest compressions:
  - Press down at least 2 inches (5 cm) with each compression. Make sure you push straight down on the victim's breastbone.
  - Deliver compressions at a rate of 100 to 120/min.
  - Allow complete chest recoil after each compression without leaning on the chest between compressions.
- Minimize interruptions in chest compressions (trying to limit any interruptions in chest compressions to less than 10 seconds).

Emphasize core concepts: Use correct hand placement, push hard and fast, allow complete chest recoil after each compression, and minimize pauses in compressions.

For all video segments, repeat the practice-while-watching segment as many times as needed for all students to complete the practice session. Observe students and provide positive and corrective feedback on their performance throughout the class.

Play Video

The video will show and discuss

Demonstration: Pocket Mask

- Ask students to position themselves at the side of their manikins to watch the demonstration.

- Tell them that they will practice using a pocket mask and complete 5 sets of 2 breaths after the demonstration.

Practice While Watching: Pocket Mask

Before playing the video, tell students to follow along with the video and complete the steps for using a pocket mask. Tell students the following:

- Position yourself at the victim's side.

- Place the pocket mask on the victim's face, using the bridge of the nose as a guide for correct position.

- Seal the pocket mask against the face.

  - Using your hand that is closer to the top of the victim's head, place the index finger and thumb along the edge of the mask that is on the nose.

  - Place the thumb of your other hand along the edge of the mask that is on the chin.

- Place the remaining fingers of your second hand along the bony margin of the jaw, and lift the jaw. Perform a head tilt–chin lift to open the airway.

- While you lift the jaw, press firmly and completely around the outside edge of the mask to seal the pocket mask against the face.

- Deliver each breath over 1 second, enough to make the victim's chest rise.

Tell students to hold the mask firmly against the face. Emphasize visible chest rise.

Play Video

The video will show and discuss

Demonstration: 1-Rescuer Adult BLS

- Ask students to position themselves at the side of their manikins to watch the demonstration.

- Tell them that they will practice the entire 1-rescuer adult BLS sequence and complete 3 sets of 30 compressions, with 2 breaths after each set of compressions after the demonstration.

Practice While Watching: 1-Rescuer Adult BLS

Before playing the video, tell students to follow along with the video. They will complete the steps for scene safety and assessment, adult compressions, and pocket mask. Refer to each skill in this lesson plan for detailed steps. Coach students to perform high-quality CPR and minimize pauses in compressions. The interval of time between breaths and compressions should be as short as possible.

Play Video

The video will show and discuss

Demonstration: Bag-Mask Device

- Ask students to position themselves at the side of their manikins to watch the demonstration.
- Tell them that they will practice using the bag-mask device and complete 5 sets of 2 breaths after the demonstration.

Practice While Watching: Bag-Mask Device

Before playing the video, tell students to follow along with the video and complete the steps for using a bag-mask device. Tell students the following:

- Position yourself directly above the victim's head.
- Place the mask on the victim's face, using the bridge of the nose as a guide for correct position.
- Use the E-C clamp technique to hold the mask in place while you lift the jaw to hold the airway open.
  - Perform a head tilt–chin lift.
  - Place the mask on the face, with the narrow portion at the bridge of the nose.
  - Use the thumb and index finger of one hand to form a C on the side of the mask, pressing the edges of the mask to the face.
  - Use the remaining fingers to lift the angles of the jaw (3 fingers form an E), open the airway, and press the face to the mask.
- Squeeze the bag to give breaths (1 second each) while watching for chest rise. Deliver each breath over 1 second, whether or not you use supplemental oxygen.
  - Instructors: Make sure students give 2 breaths and watch for chest rise.

Play Video

The video will show and discuss the following:

Demonstration: 2-Rescuer Adult BLS

- Ask students to position themselves at the side of their manikins.
- Tell them that they will practice each role of the 2-rescuer adult CPR sequence. Assign students to play Rescuer 1 and Rescuer 2.
- After the first practice-while-watching segment, the video will be repeated for students to switch and practice the duties of the other role. Each student will complete 3 sets of 30:2.

Practice While Watching: 2-Rescuer Adult BLS

Before playing the video, tell students to follow along with the video to complete the following steps:

Rescuer 1

Ask Rescuer 1 to get into position at the victim's side to practice chest compressions. The student should

- Compress the chest at least 2 inches (5 cm)
- Compress at a rate of 100 to 120/min
- Allow complete chest recoil after each compression without leaning on the chest between compressions
- Minimize interruptions in compressions (trying to limit any interruptions in chest compressions to less than 10 seconds)
- Use a compression-to-ventilation ratio of 30:2
- Count compressions out loud

Rescuer 2

Ask Rescuer 2 to get into position at the victim's head and maintain an open airway. The student should

- Perform a head tilt–chin lift or jaw thrust
- Give breaths with a bag-mask device, watching for chest rise and avoiding excessive ventilation

Tell Rescuer 2 to encourage Rescuer 1 to perform compressions that are deep enough and fast enough and to allow complete chest recoil after each compression.

Observe students and provide positive and corrective feedback on their performance.

Repeat Segment

Ask students to switch roles and repeat the practice-while-watching segment.

Lesson 3
AED for Adults, Children, and Infants   10 minutes ●

Part 1: AED Review

Part 2: AED (Students Practice)

Discussion: AED Review

Show students the AED trainer and

- Explain AED use for adults, children, and infants
- Explain how to use the AED trainer; remind students that it will not deliver a real shock
- Emphasize following the AED prompts
- Direct students to have their AED trainers out and ready to use
- Tell students that they are now going to practice using the AED

Students Practice: AED

Provide the following instructions on how to use an AED. First show the steps while using your AED trainer, and then ask students to practice.

Instructions for Students

1. Open the carrying case. Power on the AED if needed.
   - Some devices will power on automatically when you open the lid or case.
   - Follow the AED prompts for the next steps.
2. Attach AED pads to the victim's bare chest.
   - Choose adult pads (not child pads or a child system) for victims 8 years of age and older.
   - Peel the backing from the AED pads.
   - Attach the adhesive AED pads to the victim's bare chest. Place one pad on the manikin's upper-right chest (directly below the collarbone). Place the other pad to the side of the left nipple, with the top edge of the pad a few inches below the armpit.
   - Attach the AED connecting cables to the AED box (some are preconnected).
3. Clear the manikin and analyze the rhythm.
   - If the AED prompts you, clear the victim during analysis. Be sure no one is touching the victim, not even the rescuer in charge of giving breaths.
   - Some AEDs will tell you to push a button to allow the AED to begin analyzing the heart rhythm; others will do that automatically. The AED may take a few seconds to analyze.
   - The AED then tells you if a shock is needed.

4. If the AED advises a shock, it will tell you to clear the victim.

    –   Clear the victim before delivering the shock; be sure no one is touching the victim.

    –   Loudly state a "clear the victim" message, such as "Everybody clear" or simply "Clear."

    –   Look to be sure no one is in contact with the victim.

    –   Press the shock button.

5. The shock will produce a sudden contraction of the victim's muscles.

6. If the AED prompts that no shock is advised, or after any shock is delivered, immediately resume CPR, starting with chest compressions.

 ## Students Practice (Optional): 2-Rescuer Adult BLS With AED

-   After students complete the 2-rescuer CPR sequence in the practice-while-watching segment, tell them to incorporate the AED into their full adult CPR sequence.

    –   Follow the steps on the Adult CPR and AED Skills Testing Checklist for how to use the AED in a 2-rescuer CPR sequence.

-   Observe students and provide positive and corrective feedback, while emphasizing

    –   Arrival and activation of the AED

    –   Correct placement of the AED pads

    –   Following the AED prompts

-   Make sure all students complete the practice session.

Lesson 4
Special Considerations: Rescue Breathing

3 minutes ●

Instructor Tip

• Select a provider option to play for this lesson: in-facility or prehospital.

Play Video

The video will show and discuss

Demonstration: Rescue Breathing (Adults)

• Ask students to position themselves at the side of their manikins to watch the demonstration.

• Tell them that they will practice rescue breathing on the manikin after the demonstration.

• You may ask students to practice rescue breathing on infant manikins instead of adult manikins. If selecting this option, go to Students Practice: Rescue Breathing (Infants and Children) instead of Practice While Watching: Rescue Breathing (Adults).

Practice While Watching: Rescue Breathing (Adults)

Before playing the video, tell students to follow along with the video and complete the following steps for adult rescue breathing:

• Give 1 breath every 6 seconds.

• Give each breath over 1 second, ensuring that each breath results in visible chest rise.

• Check the pulse about every 2 minutes.

Repeat the practice-while-watching segment as many times as needed for all students to complete the practice session. Observe students and provide positive and corrective feedback on their performance.

Students Practice: Rescue Breathing (Infants and Children)

Discuss and then lead the students in practicing the following steps for providing rescue breathing for infants and children:

• Give 1 breath every 2 to 3 seconds (about 20 to 30 breaths per minute).

• Give each breath over 1 second.

• Each breath should result in visible chest rise.

• Check the pulse about every 2 minutes.

Repeat the practice segment as many times as needed for all students to complete the practice session. Observe students and provide positive and corrective feedback on their performance.

Lesson 5
High-Performance Teams Activity (Optional) 17 minutes

Learning Objective

Tell students that at the end of this lesson, they will be able to describe the importance of teams in multirescuer resuscitation.

Instructor Tips

- To engage students during discussion, ask open-ended questions that elicit students' own unique perspectives. This will help increase participation.

- When answering a question, make eye contact to acknowledge the student. Then, address the entire room. From time to time, direct your attention back to the student who asked the question.

- The Team Dynamics portion of this lesson focuses on the elements of effective team dynamics, including the roles everyone must play. The High-Performance Teams portion of the lesson focuses on the skills needed to achieve specific performance metrics, including a high CCF.

- CCF is the proportion of time that rescuers perform chest compressions during CPR. Shorter duration of interruptions in chest compressions is associated with better outcome. A CCF of at least 60% increases the likelihood of return of spontaneous circulation, shock success, and survival to hospital discharge. With good teamwork, rescuers can often achieve 80% CCF. In a 10-minute scenario, total chest compression time must be about 8 minutes to achieve an 80% CCF.

- Explain that BLS providers are responsible for performing only the roles on a resuscitation team that are within their training and scope of practice. It is important, however, to understand all team roles to be an effective team member.

- Select a provider option to play for this lesson: in-facility or prehospital.

- To review this lesson, students can refer to Part 5: Team Dynamics in the provider manual.

Play Video: High-Performance Teams Activity

The video will show and discuss the high-performance teams activity.

Instructor Tips

- During this activity, watch the performance of multiple rescuers simultaneously. Take note of team performance that can be improved to inform topics of discussion during the debriefing. You will present one 10-minute scenario and follow with a 5-minute debriefing.

- While students practice, you will calculate the CCF.

How Do I Measure CCF?

Option 1: Use 2 stopwatches.

1. Start one stopwatch as soon as you give the scenario to the team. Let it run continuously to the 10-minute mark (total resuscitation time) as a reminder to stop the case.

2. Use a second stopwatch to measure total compression time during the scenario. Start the stopwatch each time a Compressor starts chest compressions. Pause the stopwatch when the Compressor stops or when chest compressions are interrupted. Do this for each set of compressions during the entire scenario. Don't reset the stopwatch during the scenario; allow the stopwatch to continue counting up. This will give you the cumulative time that chest compressions were being performed during the scenario.

3. Convert the time on the second stopwatch to seconds (eg, 8 minutes = 480 seconds).

4. Divide the total compression time in seconds by the total resuscitation time in seconds (ie, 10 minutes = 600 seconds).

5. This will give you the CCF. For example, if time on the second stopwatch is 520 seconds, divide by 600 (total resuscitation time): 520/600=0.8667. Then, round to 2 places and convert to a percentage: 87%.

Option 2: Use the AHA's Full Code Pro app. This app is a free, easy-to-use, mobile application that allows rescuers to document critical interventions during CPR. You can use Full Code Pro during real resuscitation events or in practice scenarios. Go to **https://itunes.apple.com/us/app/full-code-pro/id589451064?mt=8** to download the app for iOS devices. A Full Code Pro Tutorial video is available on the AHA Instructor Network.

Option 3: Use a manikin that captures resuscitation data.

Video Pauses

- Divide students into groups for the scenario. Assign team roles. Explain that after you read the scenario, students will begin the high-performance teams activity, which will run for 10 minutes. You will evaluate the resuscitation, looking for high-quality CPR and ensuring that students enforce the principles of highly effective teams. Briefly remind students that you will be tracking CCF because limiting interruptions in chest compressions improves outcome.

- Begin CCF tracking as soon as the Compressor begins chest compressions during CPR.

Students Practice

Read this scenario to each team:

- "As part of a multirescuer emergency response team, you respond to a call about a 65-year-old woman who suddenly collapsed. Your team arrives within seconds after the incident, and you notice that a bystander is performing compression-only CPR."

- Coach students in teamwork throughout the activity. Monitor CPR performance to inform high-quality CPR coaching, including minimizing pauses in compressions during the use of the AED. Provide focused practice as needed.

- Pay particular attention to the Compressor's performance toward the end of each 2-minute rotation. Monitor for high-quality compressions of adequate rate and depth. Remind the Compressor to allow complete chest recoil after each compression without leaning on the chest between compressions.

Discussion: High-Performance Teams Activity Debriefing

- At the end of the scenario, debrief by asking team members what they thought went well and what could have been better.
  - Disclose the CCF and discuss any strategies for improvement.
  - Talk about whether the team maintained high-quality CPR.
  - Allow the team to lead the conversation; ask open-ended questions to facilitate discussion.
- Coach on improving communication with closed-loop communication principles:
  - The Team Leader gives a message, an order, or an assignment to a team member.
  - The team member gives a clear response and makes eye contact to confirm that they heard and understood the message.
  - The Team Leader listens for confirmation of task performance from the team member before assigning another task.

Skills Test (Optional)

You have the option to administer the Adult CPR and AED Skills Test now. If you choose to administer the skills test now, refer to Lesson 10: Skills Test in the HeartCode BLS Lesson Plans. Remember that you may need the adult manikins for Lesson 6: 2-Rescuer Child CPR.

Lesson 5A
Local Protocols Discussion (Optional)

20 minutes ●

Instructor Tips

- Across the country, EMS systems develop treatment protocols based on local need, preference of administration, and medical direction. In some cases, these protocols differ from established national standards, so this course may occasionally direct providers to act in ways that are not consistent with their local protocols. The AHA does not want to conflict with established local protocols.

- When you lead this discussion, make sure you know what the local protocols are. If you are a member of the local EMS system, you should already be aware of local protocols, but if you are not, study them before the course so that you can have a meaningful discussion.

Although the AHA does not endorse a particular protocol or strategy, it does issue evidence-based guidelines, which are relevant and broadly applicable. These guidelines are developed by experts in the field, who use a rigorous, scientific process. This discussion is a chance for students to articulate and practice AHA skills within the context of their local protocols.

Discussion

Lead students through a discussion about high-performance teams and local protocols. Use these questions to help guide this discussion:

- Does your system currently use a high-performance team approach to resuscitation?

- How can you incorporate high-performance teamwork into your department's protocols?

- What are some potential challenges to incorporating high-performance teamwork into your protocols?

- What are some potential challenges to high-performance teamwork in terms of location, patients, or equipment?

- How does the local protocol compare and contrast with the AHA BLS Healthcare Provider Adult Cardiac Arrest Algorithm?

The following examples show some common differences between local protocols and what is taught in the course. Use these sections only if students ask questions about these examples.

What to say when local protocols for chest compressions differ from what the course teaches:

In the course, you learned to do 30 high-quality chest compressions and then 2 breaths. This could differ from your local protocol, which may have you do 90 seconds of continuous chest compressions or 200 chest compressions before beginning breaths, or a variation of these.

- Follow the local protocol.

- The important factors in this lesson are to perform the compressions at a rate of 100 to 120/min, at least 2 inches in depth, while allowing the chest to recoil completely after each compression.

- The next Compressor should be immediately ready to switch roles to minimize interruption in compressions.

Studies show that patients who receive chest compressions at a rate of 100 to 120/min and a CCF of greater than 80% have a much better chance of survival.

What to say when local protocols for AED use differ from what the course teaches:

In the course, you learned to use the AED immediately after it arrives. This could differ from your local protocol, which may have you use the AED only after you do 200 chest compressions (or 2 minutes of CPR) or a variation of this.

- Follow the local protocol.
- Continue high-quality chest compressions up to the point of allowing the AED to analyze.
- Immediately begin chest compressions after a shock is delivered or the AED states, "no shock advised."
- Keep in mind that as time to defibrillation increases, the chance of survival decreases.

The greatest chance of survival from cardiac arrest is found when a patient receives high-quality CPR and early defibrillation.

What to say when local protocols for role assignment differ from what the course teaches:

In the course, you learned about the different roles that prehospital providers may have (Compressor, Timer/Recorder, etc). This could differ from your workplace protocol, which assigns you a role based on your role on the fire engine, ambulance, or other team.

- Follow the local protocol.
- Know your potential assignments ahead of time to reduce confusion during a real event.
- Make sure that all roles and responsibilities are clear so that interruptions in chest compressions are minimized and teamwork is smooth and efficient.
- It is critical that high-performance teams practice in the same way that they will perform in real situations.
- Appoint a Team Leader who oversees the event, assesses the efficacy of efforts, and makes changes when resuscitation performance is less than adequate.
- To optimize efforts in the future, provide a debriefing after each course scenario and after each real resuscitation attempt.

What to say when local protocols for the use of a bag-mask device differ from what the course teaches:

In the course, you learned about providing ventilation with a bag-mask device. Your local protocol may call for chest compressions only, 200 chest compressions before breaths, use of a bag-mask device with a face mask for a short time until a supraglottic airway can be placed (as soon as possible), or a variation of these.

- Follow the local protocol.
- Provide only enough volume with each ventilation to make the chest rise (do not deliver large breaths that can potentially inhibit venous blood flow back into the chest).
- When delivering ventilation during CPR with an advanced airway, provide 10 breaths per minute (excessive ventilation can increase intrathoracic pressure, impede venous return, and potentially reduce cerebral blood flow).
- Do not interrupt chest compressions for extended lengths of time to place an advanced or supraglottic airway.

Learning Objective

Tell students that at the end of this lesson, they will be able to perform high-quality CPR for a child.

Instructor Tips

- Remind students to use their mobile phones to activate the emergency response system, if applicable.
- If you are using adult manikins for the child CPR practice, inform students that they may need to use 2 hands while performing CPR because it's difficult to compress the adult manikin with 1 hand.
- Remind students that the technique used for child CPR will depend on the size of the child and the physical ability of the person performing compressions.
- Select a provider option to play for this lesson: in-facility or prehospital.

Play Video

The video will show and discuss

Demonstration: 2-Rescuer Child CPR

- Ask students to position themselves at the side of their manikins to watch the demonstration.
- Tell them that they will practice each role of the 2-rescuer child CPR sequence after the demonstration. Assign which student will play Rescuer 1 and which student will play Rescuer 2.

Practice While Watching: 2-Rescuer Child CPR

Before playing the video, tell students to follow along with the video and complete the following steps:

Rescuer 1

- Ask Rescuer 1 to get into position at the victim's side to practice chest compressions. The student should
  - Compress at least one third the depth of the chest, approximately 2 inches (5 cm)
  - Compress at a rate of 100 to 120/min
  - Allow complete chest recoil after each compression without leaning on the chest between compressions
  - Minimize interruptions in compressions (try to limit any interruptions in chest compressions to less than 10 seconds)
  - Use a compression-to-ventilation ratio of 15:2
  - Count compressions out loud

Rescuer 2

- Ask Rescuer 2 to get into position at the victim's head and maintain an open airway. The student should
    - Perform a head tilt–chin lift or jaw thrust
    - Give breaths with a bag-mask device, watching for chest rise and avoiding excessive ventilation
- Tell Rescuer 2 to encourage Rescuer 1 to perform compressions that are deep enough and fast enough and to allow complete chest recoil after each compression.
- Emphasize the core concepts: push hard, push fast; allow complete chest recoil after each compression; when giving breaths, watch for chest rise; minimize interruptions in compressions (trying to limit any interruptions in chest compressions to less than 10 seconds).

Repeat Segment

- Ask students to switch roles and repeat the practice-while-watching segment.
- Repeat the practice-while-watching segment as many times as needed for all students to complete the practice session. Each student will complete 3 sets of 15:2.

Lesson 7
Infant BLS

15 minutes ●

Part 1: Infant Compressions

Part 2: Bag-Mask Device for Infants

Part 3: 2-Rescuer Infant CPR

Learning Objective

Tell students that at the end of this lesson, they will be able to perform high-quality CPR for an infant.

Instructor Tip

- Select a provider option to play for this lesson: in-facility or prehospital.

Play Video

The video will show and discuss

Demonstration: Infant Compressions

- Ask students to position themselves at the side of their manikins to watch the demonstration.

- Tell them that they will practice infant chest compressions and will complete 3 sets of 30 compressions after the demonstration.

●

Practice While Watching: Infant Compressions

Before playing the video, tell students to follow along with the video and complete the steps for infant compressions. Tell students the following:

- Place the infant on a firm, flat surface.

- Place 2 fingers in the center of the infant's chest, just below the nipple line, on the lower half of the breastbone. Do not press the tip of the breastbone.

- Push hard and fast at a depth of at least one third the depth of the chest, approximately 1½ inches (4 cm). Deliver compressions at a rate of 100 to 120/min.

- Allow complete chest recoil after each compression without leaning on the chest between compressions.

- Minimize interruptions in compressions (trying to limit any interruptions in chest compressions to less than 10 seconds).

Tell students the following: For all video segments, repeat the practice-while-watching segment as many times as needed for all students to complete the practice session. Observe students and provide positive and corrective feedback on their performance throughout the class.

●

Play Video

The video will show and discuss

Demonstration: Bag-Mask Device for Infants

- Ask students to position themselves at the side of their manikins to watch the demonstration.
- Tell them that they will practice using the bag-mask device for infants and will complete 5 sets of 2 breaths for each student after the demonstration.

Practice While Watching: Bag-Mask Device for Infants

Before playing the video, tell students to follow along with the video and complete the steps for using a bag-mask device for infants. Tell students the following:

- Position yourself directly above the victim's head.
- Place the mask on the victim's face, using the bridge of the nose as a guide for correct position.
- Use the E-C clamp technique to hold the mask in place while you lift the jaw to hold the airway open.
  - Perform a head tilt–chin lift.
  - Place the mask on the face, with the narrow portion at the bridge of the nose.
  - Use the thumb and index finger of one hand to form a C on the side of the mask, pressing the edges of the mask to the face.
  - Use the remaining fingers to lift the angles of the jaw (3 fingers form an E), open the airway, and press the face to the mask.
- Squeeze the bag to give breaths (1 second each) while watching for chest rise. Deliver each breath over 1 second, whether or not you use supplemental oxygen.
  - Make sure students give 2 breaths and watch for chest rise.
- Repeat the practice-while-watching segment as many times as needed for all students to complete the practice session.

Play Video

The video will show and discuss

Demonstration: 2-Rescuer Infant CPR

- Ask students to position themselves at the side of their manikins to watch the demonstration.
- Tell students that they will practice each role of the 2-rescuer infant CPR sequence after the demonstration. Assign which student will play Rescuer 1 and which student will play Rescuer 2.
- After the first practice-while-watching segment, the video will repeat for students to switch and practice the duties of the other role. Each student will complete 3 sets of 15:2.

Practice While Watching: 2-Rescuer Infant CPR

Before playing the video, tell students to follow along with the video to complete the following actions:

Rescuer 1

Ask Rescuer 1 to get into position by the victim's feet to practice the 2 thumb–encircling hands technique for providing chest compressions:

- Compress at least one third the depth of the infant's chest, approximately 1½ inches (4 cm).
- Compress at a rate of 100 to 120/min.
- Allow complete chest recoil after each compression without leaning on the chest between compressions.
- Minimize interruptions in compressions (trying to limit any interruptions in chest compressions to less than 10 seconds).
- Use a compression-to-ventilation ratio of 15:2.
- Count compressions out loud.

Rescuer 2

Have Rescuer 2 get into position at the victim's head and maintain an open airway. The student should

- Perform a head tilt–chin lift or jaw thrust
- Give breaths with a bag-mask device, watching for chest rise and avoiding excessive ventilation

Tell Rescuer 2 to encourage Rescuer 1 to perform compressions that are deep enough and fast enough and to allow complete chest recoil after each compression. Emphasize core concepts: push hard, push fast; allow complete chest recoil after each compression; when giving breaths, watch for chest rise; minimize interruptions in compressions (try to limit any interruptions in chest compressions to less than 10 seconds).

Repeat Segment

Ask students to switch roles and repeat the practice-while-watching segment.

Students Practice: Infant High-Performance Teams Activity (Optional)

For additional student practice with high-performance teams, students can now complete the high-performance teams activity by using an infant scenario. Refer to Lesson 5: High-Performance Teams in the HeartCode BLS Lesson Plans for further detail on how to complete this activity with the following scenario:

"As part of a multirescuer emergency response team, you respond to a call from a parent who says her 9-month-old infant started having breathing difficulties after feeding."

Lesson 8
Relief of Choking

8 minutes

Part 1: Adult and Child Choking

Part 2: Infant Choking

Learning Objectives

Tell students that at the end of this lesson, they will be able to

- Describe the technique for relief of foreign-body airway obstruction for an adult or a child
- Describe the technique for relief of foreign-body airway obstruction for an infant

Instructor Tips

- Select a provider option to play for this lesson: in-facility or prehospital.
- To review this lesson, students can review Part 11: Choking Relief for Adults, Children, and Infants in the online course provider manual.

Discussion

Review adult and child choking with students by asking the following:

- What is the difference between mild and severe airway block?
  - Mild airway block: The person
    - Can talk or make sounds
    - Can cough loudly
  - Severe airway block: The person
    - Cannot breathe, talk, or make sounds, or
    - Has a cough that has no sound, or
    - Makes the choking sign
- What is the universal sign for choking?
  - Holding the neck with one or both hands
- Where should you give thrusts for a severely choking adult?
  - Slightly above the belly button for abdominal thrusts
  - For a large or pregnant person or a person in a wheelchair: on the lower half of the breastbone for chest thrusts
- Why is it important not to perform a blind finger sweep in a choking person?
  - The object could become lodged farther back in the airway.
- Where should you give thrusts for a severely choking child?
  - Slightly above the belly button for abdominal thrusts
  - For a large child: on the lower half of the breastbone for chest thrusts

- What is different about your body position when you give thrusts to a child vs when you give thrusts to an adult?
  - You may need to kneel to perform thrusts on a child, because of the child's size.

If students would like to practice their hand placement for abdominal thrusts for the relief of choking in an adult, students can place their hands on themselves while you watch and confirm hand placement.

Play Video

The video will show and discuss

Demonstration: Relief of Choking in a Responsive Infant

- Ask students to position themselves to watch the demonstration.
- Tell them they will practice the relief of choking on a responsive infant and will complete 1 set of 5 back slaps and 5 chest thrusts after the demonstration.

Practice While Watching: Relief of Choking in a Responsive Infant

Before playing the video, tell students to follow along with the video and complete the steps for relief of choking in a responsive infant. Tell students the following:

- Kneel or sit with the infant in your lap.
- If you can do it easily, remove clothing from the infant's chest.
- Hold the infant facedown, with the head slightly lower than the chest, resting on your forearm. Support the infant's head and jaw with your hand. Avoid compressing the soft tissues of the infant's throat. Rest your forearm on your lap or thigh to support the infant.
- Using the heel of your hand, deliver up to 5 back slaps forcefully between the infant's shoulder blades. Deliver each slap with enough force to dislodge the foreign body.
- After delivering up to 5 back slaps, place your free hand on the infant's back, supporting the back of the infant's head with the palm of your hand. The infant will be cradled adequately between your 2 forearms, with the palm of one hand supporting the face and jaw while the palm of the other hand supports the back of the infant's head.
- Turn the infant over while carefully supporting the head and neck. Hold the infant faceup, with your forearm resting on your thigh. Keep the infant's head lower than the trunk.
- Provide up to 5 quick downward chest thrusts in the middle of the chest, over the lower half of the breastbone (the same as for chest compressions during CPR). Deliver chest thrusts at a rate of about 1 per second with enough force to dislodge the foreign body.
- Repeat the sequence of up to 5 back slaps and up to 5 chest thrusts until the object is removed or the infant becomes unresponsive.
  - If the infant becomes unresponsive, activate the emergency response system. Start CPR with the additional step of checking the airway for a foreign object after each set of compressions.

Repeat the practice-while-watching segment as many times as needed for all students to complete the practice session. Observe students and provide positive and corrective feedback on their performance.

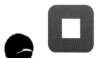

Stop Video

Ask students to return to their seats for the conclusion of the course.

Lesson 9
Conclusion

 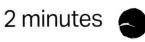

Instructor Tips

- When summarizing what was covered in the course, allow students to lead the discussion. Ask 1 or 2 students what they observed or learned during the course.

- Explain to students the importance of skills practice on an ongoing basis. Evidence shows that when providers take standardized resuscitation courses, whether online or in person, their skills decay over time. Give students clear directions on specific actions to take for further study, including AHA resources for postclassroom training.

 Discussion

To conclude the course, discuss the following with students:

- Thank students for their participation.

- Summarize what students learned during the course. Refer to the HeartCode BLS Outline in Part 3: Teaching the Course.

- Ask students if they have any questions before skills testing.

- Remember: Students taking HeartCode BLS will complete their evaluation form during the online portion of the course, before the classroom portion.

Lesson 10
Skills Test

40 minutes

Optional: This Adult CPR and AED Skills Test also can be completed at the end of Lesson 5: High-Performance Teams in the HeartCode BLS Lesson Plans.

Part 1: Adult CPR and AED Skills Test

Part 2: Infant CPR Skills Test

Instructor Tips

- For skills testing, be prepared and organized by reviewing the skills testing checklists before class. Have all materials ready to properly test students on every step.

- Make sure students review the skills testing checklist before skills testing.

Discussion

Before the Adult CPR and AED Skills Test, read the following script aloud to each student or to the whole class at once:

"This test is like a real emergency: you should do whatever you think is necessary to save the victim's life. You will have to determine for yourself what you need to do. For example, if you check for a response on the manikin and there is no response, then you should do whatever you would do for a person who is not responding. I will read a short scenario to you, but I can't answer any questions. You can treat me like another healthcare provider who has arrived with you and tell me to do something to help you. If you make a mistake or forget to do something important, don't stop. Just do your best to correct the error. Continue doing what you would do in an actual emergency until I tell you to stop. Do you have any questions before we start?"

Skills Test

- Refer to the Adult CPR and AED Skills Testing Checklist in Part 4: Testing for directions on how to test students on adult BLS skills. Check off each skill as the student demonstrates competency per the critical skills descriptors.

- After starting, if the student asks any questions about BLS skills or sequences, do not answer. Rather, tell the student, "Do what you think is best right now." If the student asks questions about what to do with the manikin, say, "Check the manikin yourself and do what you think is needed to save a life." If the student seems unsure, reiterate that he or she will be assessing the manikin and doing whatever is necessary.

Discussion

Before the Infant CPR Skills Test, read the following script aloud to the student or to all students at once:

"This test is like a real emergency: you should do whatever you think is necessary to save the victim's life. You will have to determine for yourself what you need to do. For example, if you check the response on the manikin and there is no response, then you should do whatever you would do for a person who is not responding. I will read a short scenario to you, but I can't answer any questions. You can treat me like another healthcare provider who has arrived with you and tell me to do something to help you. If you make a mistake or forget to do something important, don't stop. Just do your best to correct the error. Continue doing what you would do in an actual emergency until I tell you to stop. Do you have any questions before we start?"

Skills Test

- Refer to the Infant CPR Skills Testing Checklist in Part 4: Testing for directions on how to test students on infant BLS skills. Check off each skill as the student demonstrates competency per the critical skills descriptors.

- After starting, if the student asks any questions about BLS skills or sequences, do not answer. Rather, tell the student, "Do what you think is best right now." If the student asks questions about what to do with the manikin, tell the student, "Check the manikin yourself and do what you think is needed to save a life." If the student seems unsure, reiterate that he or she will be assessing the manikin and doing whatever is necessary.

Remediation

For students who need remediation, follow these steps, and refer to Lesson 11: Remediation in the HeartCode BLS Lesson Plans:

- Determine where the student is having trouble during their Adult CPR and AED Skills Test and/or Infant CPR Skills Test.

- If needed, replay sections of video or practice skills to reinforce learning.

- Retest skills as necessary.

- Some students may need additional practice or to repeat the course to demonstrate skills competency and receive a course completion card.

Lesson 11
Remediation

Instructor Tips

- Use the formal remediation lesson if a student did not pass the skills testing during the course.
- For further detail on remediation and retesting students, refer to Part 1: General Concepts.
- As an instructor, you will need to determine which section of the course the student is having trouble with.

 ## Play Video: Skills Testing Remediation

- Replay instruction and/or practice-while-watching segments of the video as needed to reinforce learning and for the student to have additional practice.
- Repeat practice until the student feels comfortable and is ready to move forward with the skills test.
  - Some students may need additional practice or to repeat the course to demonstrate skills competency and receive a course completion card.
- Formal remediation should occur if all boxes on the skills testing checklist are not checked as complete.

 ## Skills Test

- Retest BLS skills as necessary by using the skills testing checklists. Refer to Lesson 10 in the HeartCode BLS Lesson Plans for additional instructions on administering the skills tests.

Postcourse
Immediately After the Course

At the end of each class:

- Collect, organize, and check all course paperwork for completeness.
- Rearrange the room.
- Clean and store equipment.
- Fill out Training Center course report forms.
- Read and consider comments from course evaluations.
- Conduct a debriefing with assisting staff.
- Issue eCards according to Training Center policy. If you are unsure of the policy, check with the Training Center Coordinator.
  - Reminder: Student course completion cards must be issued to students within 20 business days after completing a class. You must submit the paperwork to your Training Center after the completion of the course for cards to be sent to students within this time frame.